TREATING FOOD ALLERGIES WITH MODERN MEDICINE

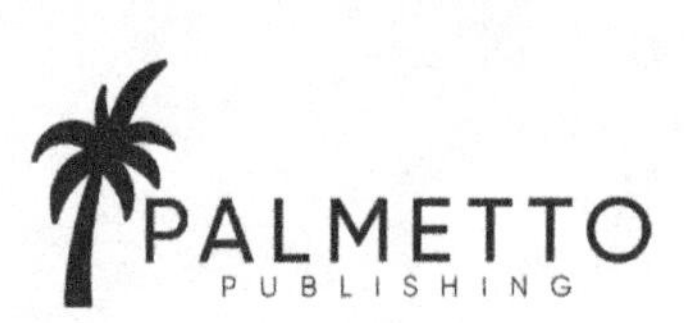

Charleston, SC
www.PalmettoPublishing.com

Treating Food Allergies with Modern Medicine
Copyright © 2021 by Elizabeth A. Muller, Elizabeth Hawkins, PhD, MPH, Sanjeev Jain, MD, PhD
All rights reserved

No portion of this book may be reproduced, stored in a retrieval system, or transmitted in any form by any means–electronic, mechanical, photocopy, recording, or other–except for brief quotations in printed reviews, without prior permission of the author.

Hardcover: 979-8-88590-020-1
Paperback: 979-8-88590-021-8
eBook: 979-8-88590-022-5

TREATING Food Allergies WITH Modern Medicine

Elizabeth A. Muller

Elizabeth Hawkins, PhD, MPH

Sanjeev Jain, MD, PhD

Table of Contents

Foreword

In 2007, a longtime patient of mine, a fourteen-year-old boy, came to me after he had just spent his vacation in the hospital, being treated for anaphylaxis. He had a known history of severe allergy to tree nuts, he was well trained in avoidance of tree nuts, and he carried his EpiPen at all times. While we didn't know for sure how he had been exposed to the tree nuts, our best guess is that it was cross contamination from a salad bar. This was his sixth anaphylactic reaction in one year. He said that "this avoidance thing isn't working out so well for me."

This young man was frustrated with food allergy avoidance and wanted to know if there was anything that we could do to treat his allergy so that he wouldn't have to be so fearful and careful. Teenagers and young adults, in particular, have a hard time with strict allergen avoidance, as well as the constraints that it puts on their social lives.

I told him that there had been a recent study on a process called oral immunotherapy for peanuts, and I had just heard a lecture from one of the authors of the study in an allergy meeting. The process of gradually building tolerance for allergens seemed to work well, and there was no reason to think that tree nut desensitization couldn't work just as well as peanut. That said, multiple tree nut desensitization had never been studied in a formal setting, and to the best of my knowledge, he would be the first patient to attempt it.

The young man told me that he was a *Star Trek* fan, and that he was ready to "boldly go where no man has gone before." His parents agreed that allergy avoidance wasn't working, and after considerable discussion of the risks and potential benefits of treatment, we decided to begin desensitization for multiple tree nuts. I was not aware of another medical doctor offering food desensitization treatment in private practice at that time, and I believe we were the first to do combined tree nuts in a single protocol. In the protocol we developed, we mixed crushed tree nuts in grape jelly using a blender, started with microscopic quantities of this mixture, and gradually over several months increased the dose. Although there were many hurdles during the process and on many occasions, our patient and his parents had second thoughts about continuing, he finally reached the maintenance dose of one gram of each nut without reacting to it. With the success of this treatment, over time, he was able to freely eat nuts without any adverse reaction. With his life-threatening condition, he would not have qualified to join the military, but after the treatment, he was able to join the naval academy and become a naval officer.

The original research on the safety and efficacy of peanut OIT was presented at the 2007 meeting of the American Academy of Allergy, Asthma and Immunology (AAAAI) by Dr. Wesley Burks and colleagues from Duke University School of Medicine and Dr. Stacie Jones and colleagues from The University of Arkansas School of Medicine. Dr. Burks has since received considerable recognition for his work on OIT, including election as the president of AAAAI in 2012.

The protocols that medical doctors, myself included, have developed over the past decade to desensitize patients to food allergies are loosely based on this early study. That said, each of us have also learned from the practice of treating patients, and there are some differences in our protocols. I think that the differences reflect the robustness of the process; oral immunotherapy works remarkably well. That said, it can be challenging for many patients, especially those who are highly sensitive. The fact that there are now over a hundred medical doctors offering oral immunotherapy in private practice is a testament to its efficacy. It also reflects the desperate need of patients, who suffer from a life of strict allergen avoidance. Even with a restricted life of food allergen avoidance, accidental exposure still happens all too often.

Since the life-transformative treatment performed on the fourteen-year old boy fourteen years ago, we have performed thousands of OIT treatments. We have desensitized patients to every food imaginable from nuts to milk, soy to buckwheat, and shrimp to cinnamon.

I remain fascinated by the latest research on the immunology of allergic diseases. In addition to oral immunotherapy patients, I have treated patients with sublingual immunotherapy (SLIT), and epicutaneous immunotherapy, or the "patch desensitization." All have their own limitations and benefits, which we have learned through experience and theoretical considerations. Using an integrated approach to desensitization by incorporating every modality and formulating a custom protocol for each patient, one can achieve a very high success rate. I go to every major allergy conference and maintain an academic interest in the theory of immunological mechanisms of desensitization; I also eagerly read the allergy journals. I incorporate all of the most recent findings in my treatment protocols. It is wonderful to be helping people in such a real and meaningful way.

Elizabeth Muller and her kids were patients of mine from 2015 to 2017—the kids for their food and environmental allergies and Elizabeth for her environmental allergies. Elizabeth wanted to deeply understand the process of food allergy treatment and frequently took notes during her consultations with me. I was impressed with her ability to understand the science and to ask questions about how we might adapt protocols to best meet her family's needs. She was willing to accept a degree of informed risk and she asked about the potential risks of dropping the rest period during oral immunotherapy, updosing at home for her son, and moving toward every other day dosing even before her daughter's blood test suggested sustained tolerance.

While Elizabeth and her kids were in treatment with me, the buzz about food allergy treatments began spreading rapidly, due primarily to word of mouth and social media. Elizabeth was part of this process and one of the creators of several social media groups, including a Facebook group for parents of patients in treatment with me. More and more new patients mentioned to my staff that they were starting treatment because they had heard about it from Elizabeth. She was clearly an influencer when it came to getting the word out.

During one of our consultations, Elizabeth mentioned her frustration with the lack of high-quality information on food allergy treatments.

She pointed out that most parents have a hard time making sense of the scientific papers and that social media is not an authoritative source of information. Once her children had completed treatment, she mentioned that she wanted to do something about this and suggested that we coauthor a book on food allergy treatments. She wanted the book to be aimed at parents, and she wanted it to cover *all* treatment methods that are currently available. Her words echoed something that I had been feeling myself for quite some time, and I immediately agreed.

This book is meant for anyone who would like to know more about food allergy treatments—their benefits, risks, and the process of treatment. The scientific information included here is based on detailed interviews with me. I have medically vetted all the information in this book and stand behind everything that is said. I sincerely hope that this work will provide families with a reliable source of information on some of the most important new medical treatments of our generation. —Sanjeev Jain, MD, PhD

Introduction

On Wednesday November 19, 2014, I got a call from my eleven-month-old son's daycare. The director thought my son Asim was having an allergic reaction, and while she didn't think it was anaphylaxis, she thought I might like to come see for myself. Was I nearby? Fortunately, I worked just a block away from the daycare facility, and I ran there as fast as I could. By the time I arrived, his reaction had progressed to full-blown anaphylaxis. It was obvious to me that he needed emergency epinephrine.

He had never been prescribed an EpiPen. Thankfully, however, I had one in my purse that was prescribed for his older sister. You see, this wasn't my first experience with food allergies. That frightening introduction had come a few years earlier when my daughter Layla had an anaphylactic reaction to playing with the shell of an egg. So with my heart racing and my hands trembling, I quickly dug out the epinephrine injector and stabbed my son in his thigh. Then I rushed him to the hospital.

An hour later, as they monitored him in the emergency room, I had time to reflect on what had just happened. He had been diagnosed with Food Protein-Induced Enterocolitis Syndrome (FPIES) to cow and soy milk, but he had not ingested either of these and was not considered at risk for anaphylaxis. I had grown used to the idea of having one severely allergic child (his sister), but could I handle *two*? And how was this even possible? I had taken all of the recommended steps to help prevent food allergies with him (vaginal birth, breastfeeding, early exposure to allergens, etc.).

It wasn't until several months later that we truly began to understand the full extent of his severe food allergies, and that was when the devastation hit. Not only was he severely anaphylactic to milk (and all dairy products), but he was also allergic to every seed, nut, and legume that we tested. Blood and skin tests are notoriously unreliable, but my son failed every oral challenge that we conducted, with only one exception (yay, coconut!). Despite valiant efforts on everyone's part, Asim had severe reactions and multiple episodes of anaphylaxis before he was barely a year old. He could not drink any of the popular infant formulas due to the presence of cow, goat, or even soy milk. He had several episodes of "mystery anaphylaxis," in which nobody could figure out what triggered the reaction because he *didn't* eat any of the foods that he was allergic to leading us to question whether some allergen was furtively wafting through the air.

I was already somewhat familiar with managing severe food allergies because my five-year-old daughter was allergic to peanuts, tree nuts, fish, and buckwheat. With her, we had followed our allergist's advice of "avoid and hope to outgrow." And she did outgrow two allergies before age four, to egg and coconut. However, year after year her other allergies became worse, not better. I later learned that this is actually more common than outgrowing nut allergies. By the time she was five, our allergist told us that some of her allergies had become so severe that she would probably never outgrow them and we needed to learn how to cope and endure.

I could fathom a challenging yet somewhat "normal" life for my daughter, despite her severe allergies. Yes, there would be social exclusion at many events. Potlucks, in particular, were virtually impossible to navigate. Harder for me was imagining her teens and twenties, when she would have to ask her boyfriend what he had for dinner before she could kiss him.

However, given the extent of my son's multiple severe allergies (milk, in particular, is absolutely everywhere), standard avoidance recommendation was not an attractive option. I could not imagine any sort of "normal" life for my little boy. I couldn't take him to social events, as bringing his own special food was not enough to keep him safe. Toddlers at parties contaminate their hands with cake frosting and other messy foods and then leave bits of these foods everywhere. Thinking ahead to preschool, I wanted to send him to the same school his sister attended, a school that I picked based on its educational approach and the quality of the teachers. I did not want to be limited to schools with the strictest food allergy policies.

When my son failed his baked milk challenge at fifteen months, I went home and cried. Baked milk allergy is a really disastrous one. Eighty percent of milk-allergic kids can tolerate baked milk. And if you can tolerate baked milk, then it will help you outgrow the milk allergy. But my son was anaphylactic to just a tiny crumb of baked muffin. Our allergist told us that it "wasn't a good sign." To me, that was a horrific understatement. Even a crumb from a piece of bread or cake could mean death. I could hardly stand thinking about the implications for his life. But I had to.

When I was done crying, I decided to take an independent look into food allergy treatments. Our allergist at that time had not been optimistic about them. A quick Google search found a few articles on possible "future cures," but nothing on treatments available then. At that time, there were no books on how to treat severe food allergies on Amazon, only a multiplicity of books on how to live with them, how to adjust your lifestyle, and how to cope and endure. But I was not ready to give up and take that path.

The scientific papers on treatments, primarily oral immunotherapy (OIT), were all behind expensive pay walls and not readily available to the public. Thankfully, I was able to use my personal and professional connections with UC Berkeley to access the articles. They were challenging to read. Even with my scientific background, it took considerable time and effort to parse what they were saying. But I kept at it.

Later, I discovered on Facebook that treatment actually was available, offered both through clinical trials (very limited and generally with long waitlists) and in private practice offices all over the United States. And I could connect with other parents whose kids were in treatment. It turns out that one of the most respected food allergy treatment doctors, Dr. Jain, has a practice only an hour's drive from our home! I chose to switch allergy care to Dr. Jain, and we started on an intense and rewarding journey of food allergy treatments. By the time my son was fifteen months old, both of my children had started treatments aimed at allowing them to live normal lives and be able to "free eat" their allergens within a few years.

As I learned and experienced more, I became determined to help other food allergies families struggling with similar issues. The aim of this book is to provide an authoritative source of information on all of the scientifically grounded treatment options that are currently available, from the point of view of a parent who has been through it. The book discusses the different treatment options and will help guide parents to pick those that are best for them. It presents the challenges, risks, and rewards of pursuing each of the treatments described. I use many personal examples drawn from my own experiences of treating my children's allergies, as well as from people I have met and talked with in person, over the phone, and online through internet forums.

I began writing *Treating Food Allergies with Modern Medicine* in close collaboration with our allergist, Dr. Jain. Over a period of about fifteen months, I had weekly meetings with him, asking him about the science of allergies and his experience with each of the treatment methods discussed in the book. Dr. Jain has been invaluable in ensuring that information included here agrees with his current scientific and medical understanding of treating food allergies while acknowledging that the pace of science is constantly advancing.

When the book was about halfway complete, my startup company, Deep Isolation, took off, and I suddenly had much less time for writing. At Dr. Jain's suggestion, I reached out to Elizabeth Hawkins, who is a food allergy mom and a child psychologist. Dr. Jain had worked with Elizabeth on the psychological challenges that some patients face when treating food allergies, so she seemed like a perfect fit to help us finish the book. To our delight, Elizabeth was intrigued by the project and willing to help out. Not only did Elizabeth help us to complete the book, but she has also added another dimension to it—that of child (and parent!) psychology. The book is richer from her contribution. While still primarily written in my voice, with the medical information provided by Dr. Jain, Elizabeth occasionally jumps in and she shares some of her personal story in chapter 12. She has also included examples from other food allergy families, greatly enriching the perspective.

Part I
Starting Your Journey

Chapter 1:

Food Allergies in Our Society

If you're reading this book, chances are you or someone you care about has food allergies and you are here trying to learn all you can in order to help them. Researchers now estimate that there are 32 million people in the United States with food allergies, including one in every ten adults and one in every thirteen children. Rates of anaphylactic food reactions increased 377 percent between 2007 and 2016. These alarming numbers have led serious scientific organizations to call food allergies an epidemic. The problem is growing faster than the community can address it.

Rise of the Epidemic

Why has this precipitous rise in food allergies occurred during the past few decades? Food allergies are part of what is known as the atopic syndrome, a constellation of disorders that also includes eczema, asthma, and environmental allergies. While it is not inevitable that one person will experience all four of these conditions, we know that they tend to cluster together. Nobody knows for sure what it causing the food allergy epidemic, but it is generally believed that both genetic and environmental factors are involved in the development of atopic diseases.

There is certainly a genetic component, as allergies (and atopic diseases more generally) can be passed on from one generation to the next. It is relatively common that identical twins will both have allergies, although not necessarily to the same foods. In one small study on peanut allergy, it was reported that 64.3 percent of identical twins both had peanut allergy as compared to 6.8 percent for fraternal twins. However, having exactly the same genes does not guarantee that both individuals will have allergies, especially if they have been raised apart in different environments.

Why do some people express those genes while some do not? Perhaps one of the most accepted theories of food allergy proliferation is the hygiene hypothesis. This posits that our environment has become too clean and that, in susceptible individuals, this can disrupt healthy development of the immune system. Humans need a diversity of microorganisms to help perform immunologic and digestive functions. Antibiotics have been massively overused in our society, through their use in soaps and sanitizers; over-prescribing and poor utilization practices for individual illness; and to control illness among animals in the food chain. Antibiotics kill both beneficial and harmful bacteria. When the gut biome is disrupted, the ingestion of an otherwise benign food can cause the immune system to mount an inflammatory allergic response.

Environmental factors occur on both a systemic and personal level. For example, we know that food allergies are more prevalent in western countries and in more urban environments. Both of these are presumed to be more sanitary and sterile and have less diversity in bacterial strains. Food allergies also occur at greater frequency in locations farther away from the equator and among children born in the fall and winter months. Americans, especially in northern climates, spend more times indoors than they previously did, and public health interventions against skin cancer have successfully increased the use of sunscreen when people are outdoors. Both of these impact vitamin D levels, and deficiencies are linked with increases in food allergies. Furthermore, in the US, it is recommended that women take prenatal vitamins with high levels of folate to reduce risk of neural tube defects. However, preliminary research suggests that super-physiologic levels of folate might be related to the development of food allergies.

On an individual level, the use of antibiotics at birth and in early childhood impacts the microbiome of the child. Other individual risk factors for food allergies include being born by C-section, not being breastfed, and the use of infant formula. Consumption of highly processed food, which is low in fiber and high in simple carbohydrates, also adversely affects gut microbiome. All of these influence what microorganisms a child is exposed to and, in genetically susceptible individuals, may cause sensitization to certain food proteins rather than tolerance.

Other Food Related Conditions

A food allergy is an immune-mediated reaction to a certain food. Most symptoms occur within minutes to two hours of ingestion. Most food allergies involve proteins in the blood called immunoglobulin E (IgE) antibodies. When someone has been sensitized to a particular food, their body creates IgE antibodies to that food's protein structure. When the food is eaten, the IgE antibodies trigger an immune system response and cause mast cells to release chemicals, including histamine. These chemicals lead to the symptoms of an allergic reaction. Symptoms can range from mild to severe. Reactions often impact multiple organs and body systems, and can be fatal.

This book is focused on food allergy treatments, but I'd like to take a moment to briefly address other food related conditions that might be mistaken for an allergy. They differ from true food allergies in important ways that have treatment implications.

Food Sensitivities/Intolerances

This is a nondescriptive term that can mean many things. Food induced immune responses may also be cell-mediated instead of antibody mediated and can lead to unwanted digestive or intestinal symptoms. A lot of factors influence food sensitivity, and reactions can be similar to mild allergies, further confusing the distinction. Dr. Jain notes that both food sensitivities and mild food allergies can cause gastrointestinal problems and even more vague symptoms like "feeling tired." Many people suffer with these complaints but do not seek the advice of an allergist. Without this, it can be challenging to determine whether a food sensitivity is actually a mild allergy, a distinction that has important ramifications for treatment.

The most common food sensitivity is lactose intolerance. Lactose intolerance is not an immunological reaction and thus cannot be treated using the methods described in this book. With lactose intolerance, the body is unable to digest the milk sugar lactose in the stomach, so it moves on to the colon. In the colon, lactose gets digested by bacteria. Other sugars and food ingredients, widely included in the FODMAP (fermentable oligo- di- and mono-saccharides and polyols) group, can also cause similar symptoms in individuals who are not able to digest them well. When certain bacteria digest lactose or FODMAP group of sugars, they release mediators that can cause gas and bloating, diarrhea, and stomach discomfort. There are enzyme treatments to promote better digestion that help some people and probiotics that could help in some cases.

Celiac Disease

Celiac disease is an autoimmune disease related to an intolerance to gluten, a protein found in wheat, rye, and barley. It is estimated to affect about 1 percent of people worldwide. When people with celiac disease eat gluten, their body mounts an immune response that attacks the small intestine, causing an inflammatory response and damage. This damage impairs the body's ability to properly absorb nutrients and causes serious health problems. Untreated, celiac disease can also lead to the development of other autoimmune disorders such as Type I diabetes, multiple sclerosis, inflammatory bowel disease, or thyroid disease.

Celiac disease is not the same as wheat allergy. While wheat allergy can be treated using the methods described in this book, celiac disease cannot. Currently, the only treatment for celiac disease is strict adherence to a gluten-free diet.

Oral Allergy Syndrome

Oral Allergy Syndrome (OAS) most typically manifests as a reaction in the mouth after eating a food. It is most commonly caused by raw fruits, raw vegetables, or raw nuts. It is usually associated with environmental allergies (e.g., hay fever), but many adults and kids with hay fever may not know that they have environmental allergies, so this should not necessarily be used for at home diagnosis.

Interestingly, OAS is not actually an allergy to the food being eaten. Rather it is a cross reaction to tree or weed pollen. The protein structure of these environmental allergens is similar to that found in certain raw foods. When the food is eaten, the immune system mistakes the food protein for the pollen protein and directs an allergic response to it. People affected with OAS can usually eat cooked forms of the same foods they react to when consumed raw. During the heating process, the protein structure is changed and the immune system no longer recognizes the food as an allergen. OAS is more common during the pollen season but can occur any time of the year. Treatment for OAS is directed at the underlying pollen allergy. Sublingual (SLIT) immunotherapy and allergy shots are both good treatment options.

Eosinophilic esophagitis

Eosinophilic esophagitis (more commonly called EoE) is a chronic allergic inflammation of the esophagus, the tube that sends food from the mouth to the stomach. In EoE, large numbers of white blood cells called eosinophils are found in the tissue of the esophagus. When eating problem foods with EoE, the esophagus can narrow to the point that food gets stuck. Common symptoms among children include coughing, a feeling that something is stuck in their throat, vomiting, and recurring abdominal pain. Teenagers and adults most often have difficulty swallowing, particularly dry or dense, solid foods. The esophagus can narrow to the point that food gets stuck, which is called food impaction, a medical emergency.

EoE is considered to be a chronic condition and is not outgrown. The standard of care is to remove identified allergens from the diet; remove all common allergens from the diet (even if standard allergy testing does not suggest a specific allergy); adhere to an elemental diet (removing all proteins from the diet); and/or using medications to reduce the number of eosinophils in the esophagus and improve symptoms (e.g., corticosteroids and proton pump inhibitors).

There is some controversy because many people theorize that OIT treatment can cause EoE. It is true that OIT may allow exposure to an allergen that had been avoided previously, and this may trigger EoE that had been dormant. But when done carefully, EoE patients can be treated with all of the methods described in this book. The main challenge with OIT is that the passage of food down the esophagus can cause additional inflammation. Some doctors have their patients swallow capsules of their allergens to avoid the food coming into contact with the throat (rather than chewing and swallowing). Others go very slowly, such that treatment can take years, as opposed to the more common months. SLIT and the patch are excellent options for EoE patients and reduce some of the risks associated with using OIT. Chinese Herbs can also be an effective treatment for EoE patients, as they reduce allergic inflammation and IgE without any swallowing of allergens involved.

Current Recommendations for Prevention and Treatment of Food Allergy

The guidance on food allergy prevention has recently done a complete turnabout, as doctors recognize the importance of exposure to foods as a means to prevent allergy. In 2003, the American Academy of Pediatrics (AAP) released a statement on prevention of food allergy in children that recommended delaying the introduction of cow's milk until one year of age; egg until two years of age; and peanut, tree nut, and fish until three years of age. This recommendation was reinforced in 2006 when the American College of Allergy, Asthma and Immunology concluded that early introduction of solid foods could increase the risk of food allergy and other atopic diseases. However, there were studies that disagreed with these recommendations, and in 2008 the AAP released new guidelines that stated that there was no evidence that delaying the introduction of solid foods beyond four to six months was protective against the development of food allergies.

Confusing, right? As this was debated in the scientific literature, in books and in doctor's offices around the country, families were being told to delay introduction of allergenic foods, especially in at-risk populations. There seemed to be no downside to being cautious and slow in starting solid foods while the risk was great. As we know, there is often a lag between the release of public-health guidelines and the impacts they have on society. We now know that, during this period of time, rates of food allergy and severe reactions among children skyrocketed.

Results of the landmark *Learning Early About Peanut* (LEAP) study were first shared in early 2015 and helped solidify a new understanding of the development of food allergy. These researchers followed 640 infants at high risk of developing peanut allergy and randomized them into two groups: peanut avoidance and regular peanut consumption. Among the children who avoided peanut, 17 percent developed peanut allergy by age five. Among the children who regularly consumed peanut product starting in infancy, only 3 percent developed peanut allergy by age five. Researchers extended their findings in the *Persistence of Oral Tolerance to Peanut* (LEAP-On) study published in 2016. They followed 556 of the original 640 children (274 previous peanut consumers and 282 previous peanut avoiders) from the LEAP study. For one year, all 556 children were asked to avoid peanut consumption. At the end of the year, 4.8 percent of the original peanut consumers were found to be allergic to peanut compared to 18.6 percent of the original peanut avoiders.

The LEAP and LEAP-On studies helped change guidelines for parents about how and when to introduce solid foods to their infants. Over time, we will see the impact this has on the rates of food allergy development. In the meantime, though, we have approximately 32 million Americans with diagnosed food allergies. What is the standard medical advice for managing and treating their allergies?

Those diagnosed with food allergies are told to strictly avoid their allergen, carry emergency epinephrine wherever they go, and hope to outgrow the allergy, especially if diagnosed in a young child. Alas, outgrowing an allergy is far less likely than many physicians seem to think. Only about 20 percent of peanut-allergic children will outgrow their allergy, and that number drops to 15 percent for tree nut allergies. Rates for fish and shellfish allergies are even lower, with only 4 to 5 percent outgrowing those. The story is better for milk and egg allergies, with about 60 to 80 percent able to eat those foods freely by age sixteen. Children with multiple allergens or asthma are generally considered less likely to outgrow allergies, and most allergists think that there is only a tiny chance of outgrowing an allergy with a very high specific IgE level.

Allergen avoidance is easier said than done. Children with food allergies suffer in countless ways. They and their families live daily with the threat of serious harm coming from ingesting or even being around common foods, something most people take for granted. Diet is obviously impacted and may lead to nutritional challenges and deficiencies. There are often restrictions in lifestyle and home/school environments, sometimes in dramatic ways, to keep kids safe. Celebrations and holidays take on a new level of fear and preparation. Allergies frequently impact choices in friends and activities. Children can become isolated and miss out on everyday joys such as playdates and parties. In addition to the physical, emotional, and social costs of food allergies is the financial cost. A national study estimates that having a child with a food allergy increases the yearly cost of raising that child by about 30 percent or $4,184 per year.

My family lived this restricted life. Our home had no milk, soy, eggs, tree nuts, peanuts, seeds, buckwheat products, beans, peas, or any other legumes. After one terrifying party experience with my son when he was eighteen months old, I stopped taking him to birthday parties and potlucks. Before treatment, he had never, not even once, been out to eat at a restaurant. We couldn't even take him to cafes with his own food because there was steamed milk wafting through the air.

Adults who interact with children with food allergies (family, teachers, camp counselors, athletic coaches, friends) need to be prepared to give epinephrine shots in the case of a reaction. Yet many caregivers find that responsibility extremely uncomfortable. They are unsure about when epinephrine is needed and question their ability to administer the shot properly. Many people avoid getting shots themselves and are afraid of handling an autoinjector needle. If you are the parent of a food-allergic child, often your primary concern about your child participating in social events is whether or not the adults involved can be trusted to keep your child safe from allergens and be prepared to handle an emergency situation should it arise. It is not surprising that many food allergy parents vet their children's friends (or rather the parents) extremely carefully.

For all these reasons and more, severe food allergies are protected as a disability by the federal government. Many parents these days use a "504 plan," which legally qualifies their child as having a disability and allows for needed accommodations in public school settings. A 504 plan may prohibit food in the child's classroom, require a "nut free" table at the cafeteria, and guarantee parental participation in field trips and special activities. But as food allergies move beyond peanuts to milk, fruits, vegetables, seeds, and more, school inclusion is getting harder and harder to implement. Food-free classrooms are an option that works for all food allergies, but they are highly unpopular with other parents, as they mean no birthday treats, no classroom activities involving food, and no celebrating special occasions such as end-of-the-year parties with food.

These are the worries food allergy parents struggle with when their child is still young enough to be largely under their influence. And then the dreaded teenage years arrive. In addition to the typical issues that come with adolescence, parents now have much less control over their children's diet, friends, and social life. And teens are more apt to take risks. Experience shows that most teens hate carrying their epinephrine injectors everywhere they go. They also hate being different and having to explain why they can't have ice cream or pizza or random snacks like everyone else. Most food allergy deaths in the United States occur in teenagers and young adults who were not carrying their auto injectors when they had an anaphylactic reaction. In 2016, a Quebec woman came forward to share the tragic story of her twenty-year-old daughter's death four years earlier. She was allergic to peanuts but had not told her boyfriend and was not carrying epinephrine. Unbeknownst to her, he had eaten a peanut butter sandwich and then brushed his teeth. She had an anaphylactic reaction after they kissed and subsequently died. Imagine trying to convince your teenager or young adult not to kiss anyone without first telling them about your food allergies and checking to see what they had eaten that day.

Sources of Information on Food Allergy Treatments

When I started researching food allergy treatments for my kids, I was frustrated that there was no official organization that provided information about the wide range of new treatments available. Instead, I went directly to the scientific literature and read the articles voraciously. These are available online to the medical and academic community, although they generally require a paid subscription or institutional affiliation. Most parents do not have access to the scientific literature or the ability to understand what are often very technical papers.

I'd like to be able to say that doctors are reliably knowledgeable about current research and can help inform their patients, but I haven't found this to be true. Dr. Jain keeps on top of the research and readily incorporates new findings into his practice. However, this wasn't the case with our other medical providers, including our previous allergist who was aware of the treatments but did not share information about them with us. Food allergy parents often find themselves in the role of educating not only family and friends but also other medical providers. For example, once my kids started treatment, I printed out and brought copies of scientific articles for my pediatrician, who had heard of the treatments and was interested in learning more.

Today there is more information available online and for free about food allergy treatment than ever before. Food Allergy Research and Education (FARE) privately funds food allergy treatment research and has helped facilitate national clinical networks and collaborations. However, they do not currently support these treatments being used outside of their network. So while their website will help you locate clinical trials, it does not help connect patients to private practice allergists who are performing large numbers of desensitization cases. Since clinical trials are not accessible to most, this leaves millions of families confused about their options.

As a result, parents have turned to groups through Facebook and built a robust support community online. The most popular food allergy treatment groups on Facebook have thousands of members, mostly parents of kids who are in treatment, have completed treatment, or who are considering treatment. There are Facebook groups for all of the main treatments discussed in this book. Most were created by parents, not doctors, and while they are extremely helpful, they are not ideal as a primary source of information.

Another helpful online resource, www.OIT101.org, was created by a mother and completed with the help of other parents of food allergic children. This website provides helpful information on OIT and case studies are available, including for my two children. The OIT101 website also has a tool that patients can use to find OIT doctors near them, though not all OIT practices are listed. While the website briefly describes other treatment options, it focuses primarily on OIT.

Chapter 2:
Introduction to Food Allergy Treatment

The standard recommendation for food allergy management has been strict avoidance, even in the case of minor reactions and/or high tolerance of the food. More recent research suggests that this may actually be compounding the problem and causing allergies to get worse, not better. We know that the number of children with allergies persisting into adulthood is increasing, giving scientists serious concern that food allergies are not only getting more common but also getting more severe.

What most parents are never told, not by their pediatrician and not even by their allergist, is that there are treatments available today to overcome food allergies. Although these are well respected in the medical community, many allergists are hesitant to offer the treatment themselves. Typically they say that they like to be "conservative" and that the treatments aren't yet ready for widespread use. They prefer to stick with the avoidance approaches they learned when they were in medical school.

Some doctors argue that changes in the approach would best wait until further studies have been done. Often that caution reflects the doctor's ignorance of how rapidly the field has advanced; it is hard to keep up-to-date while engaged in full-time practice. Some doctors say that they want to wait for "FDA approval." Ironically, although this sounds like a properly cautious approach, it actually reflects ignorance. The FDA's responsibility is limited to *drug treatments*. The FDA does not review or approve treatments that involve natural foods and are drug-free. Yet drug-free treatments are at the heart of many of the modern scientific advances.

Many doctors say that food allergy treatments are not actually a "cure" and instead advise their patients to wait for better options on the horizon. Waiting for future cures may be the right decision for some patients. Some people may learn about the treatments available today and decide that they would prefer to wait and see what happens in the future. It is possible that some of the future treatments could be easier, quicker, and with fewer risks of reactions along the way. It is even possible that there could be a quick and easy "cure" developed soon.

Any decision as to whether to treat now or wait, though, should be an informed decision, grounded in an understanding of the treatments available today, their risks, and their benefits. It should also be based on a realistic understanding of the timelines involved in upcoming treatments. While there is a chance that there could be a quick and easy permanent cure, there is also a chance that many of the future options could be just as challenging as the treatments available today. Whatever a family decides, their decisions should be based on quality information about the risks and benefits of the treatments available today and those on the horizon.

The methods I will discuss in this book are medically recognized treatments. Some of them are even covered by health insurance. Thousands of children are being effectively treated for their food allergies every year, and many can safely and freely eat the foods they previously had to fear. My own two children are in this group. The treatments have worked! It has been this wonderful success, together with the continued suffering of other parents and children who are not aware of these treatments, which leads me to write this book.

Evidence-Based Treatments

Immunotherapy involves using your food allergens to gradually retrain your immune system and build tolerance to that food. It starts with repeated exposures to tiny doses that incrementally increase over time, allowing the body to become tolerant to the allergen and thus produce less of an allergic response. This process is known as desensitization. People have used immunotherapy for hundreds of years, though today the method of delivery is somewhat more sophisticated. While we understand quite a bit about immunotherapy and the mechanisms that underlie it, there is still much to learn.

In part two of this book, I provide detailed information on four immunotherapy treatments for food allergies: Oral immunotherapy (OIT); Sublingual immunotherapy (SLIT); Epicutaneous immunotherapy (EPIT or the Patch); and Food Allergy Herbal Formula-2 (FAHF-2 or Chinese Herbs). Each of these has been established in peer-reviewed articles in prominent scientific journals. Each treatment has both a scientific evidence base as well as practice-based evidence to support it. While not yet used in mainstream allergy practices as the standard of care, these treatments are being successfully implemented across the country.

Goals of Treatment

Families pursue immunotherapy with different goals and benchmarks for success. In this book, I use the term *treatment* when talking about the process of desensitizing food allergies so that larger amounts can be safely consumed. Desensitization relies on ongoing regular exposure to the allergen for maintaining treatment gains.

The lowest level of desensitization protection is to no longer worry about cross-contamination and how food is prepared or manufactured. While continuing to strictly avoid foods that knowingly contain the allergen, you are freed from having to call manufacturers with a detailed list of questions and decide whether to allow your child to eat foods prepared in the same facility or on the same lines as foods containing the allergen.

The next level is to become "bite proof," which means your child can tolerate a single bite of their allergen without major reaction. While still actively avoiding foods that contain the allergen, you might no longer worry about those "may contain" statements on labels. And you may feel more reassured about your child eating allergen-free food prepared by friends and family or eating at restaurants. Becoming bite-proof can relieve a lot of anxiety and distress for families.

Being able to add your allergen into your diet and eat as much as you would like is known as "free eating" status. While you still rely on having a regular maintenance dose of the allergen for protection, you are free to eat as much additional allergen as you would like. Parents are able to stop reading labels completely (at least for that allergen), go out to restaurants without talking to the chef, and feel a measure of comfort letting their child roam at parties and potlucks.

Sustained tolerance is the holy grail of food allergy treatment and refers to long-term unresponsiveness to the food, regardless of how often it is consumed. In other words, the food allergy has been "cured," and there are lasting immunologic changes that make a person able to treat the food the same as someone without an allergy. Many people have gotten to this point of being cured using the treatments described in this book.

A note of caution. While there is every indication that individuals can cure an allergy and reach sustained tolerance, those predisposed to allergies can go on to develop a new allergy at some point in their life. This might be especially the case for people with multiple allergies and/or other atopic diseases. Due to this, Dr. Jain advocates for a conservative approach of continuing to carry emergency epinephrine even if the patient has reached sustained tolerance.

How Immunotherapy Works

So how and why do these treatments work? While a deep explanation is beyond the scope of this book, some detailed information will help readers understand and evaluate the treatments. Broadly speaking, the immune system has two main branches: the stimulatory arm and the regulatory arm. Both are critically important in immune system functioning, and they are designed to work together. The stimulatory arm allows our bodies to mount an immune response to fight off infection or disease, a process that is misdirected toward harmless food in those with allergies. The regulatory arm dampens the stimulatory response and allows the body to return to baseline and rest. This is one way the immune system distinguishes between benign proteins (such as pollen or proteins in our own body) and proteins originating from a virus, bacteria, or parasites.

When a person is exposed to an antigen or an allergen, the default immune response is activation of the regulatory arm, unless the immune system receives additional danger signals. These danger signals activate the stimulatory response and cause immune cells, such as T-helper cells, to release mediators, including cytokines and chemokines, which lead to development or worsening of allergic reactions. In OIT, activation of the regulatory arm occurs when the body is presented with small amounts of the allergen protein through the gastrointestinal tract. Dose is critical and highly individualized, as it needs to be large enough to activate the regulatory arm of the immune system but not so large that it causes an allergic reaction. When the amount is just right, the mast cell receptors are blocked and do not release their contents. If the dose is too high, the mast cells release their contents (such as histamine), leading to an intense allergic reaction. In addition to the allergic reaction acutely happening, this response may also activate the stimulatory arm and make allergies worse moving forward.

In the early stages of OIT, desensitization relies heavily on a mechanism called mast cell and basophil anergy. This is a process in which the cells responsible for releasing the mediators that cause an allergic reaction become unresponsive to the same amount of allergen for a short time after these cells are initially exposed to that allergen. The period during which these cells remain unresponsive is called a refractory period. Rush or rapid immunotherapy protocols take full advantage of this refractory period. In these protocols, the allergic person is reintroduced to the allergen within the refractory period in gradually escalating doses. In order for this approach to work, the IgE molecules on the mast cells need to be continuously occupied by the allergen. This is the rationale for daily dosing during treatment and maintenance phases of OIT.

Activation of the regulatory arm of the immune system typically happens through the lymph nodes and is an important mechanism for longer term desensitization in OIT. It is also a primary mechanism of desensitization in SLIT, EPIT, and FAHF-2, which do not induce anergy as OIT does. The regulatory arm is responsible for calming down the immune system and helps to dampen allergic activity. While these treatments do modulate the immune system and can prevent allergic reactions, the protection they offer can be overwhelmed by a large amount of food-specific IgE protein presented to the body. This is because the regulatory arm of the immune system does not block allergens from binding to IgE on the surface of the mast cell receptors, which are primarily responsible for an anaphylactic reaction.

Over time and with repeated consistent exposure, food allergy immunotherapy treatments have the potential to lead to sustained tolerance. One mechanism for achieving this is generation of IgG4 molecules. This class of antibodies can bind allergens but unlike IgE, they cannot activate an allergic reaction. For this reason, when the body makes enough IgG4 antibodies against the allergen, they are able to compete with IgE and prevent allergic reactions. Another mechanism for reaching sustained tolerance is apoptosis—or programmed cell death. When this occurs, allergy producing cells are eliminated from the body, and IgE levels fall sharply.

Effectiveness of Immunotherapy

The food allergy treatments described in this book demonstrate varying levels of effectiveness, which will be covered in detail in Part Two. When treatment and maintenance protocols are followed, they tend to work, meaning patients receive some level of desensitization to their allergen. While I am here to share my story and those of others who have had success, I do want to acknowledge that pursing treatment is not for every family.

There are many people who start and then discontinue treatment. One of the reasons that people drop out is that they don't fully appreciate the challenges of following treatment protocols. Treatment can be time consuming, logistically challenging, expensive, and in many cases require parents to become their own advocates and treatment experts. Minor allergic reactions during treatment are fairly common. Serious reactions are less common but still do occur. The risk of these reactions frightens parents. Families are often overloaded with other commitments or are struggling with other health concerns. Our medical system is ill-equipped to support the needs of patients, and there are few official resources for parents to turn to for help. All of these are real and valid obstacles to participating in treatments.

Treatments to Avoid

If you've been researching treatments for food allergies, you've no doubt run into one or more of the interventions listed here. These approaches might have popular support but are not backed by scientific evidence and should be avoided as food allergy treatments.

Elimination Diets

An elimination diet is a structured plan for avoiding foods or groups of foods suspected of causing reactions in an individual. After a period of avoidance, each food is reintroduced into the diet so we can see which might be causing symptoms. While elimination diets may be helpful for detecting food sensitivities or intolerances, they do not work for anaphylactic food allergies. In fact, they may make things worse. By eliminating foods from your diet, you may decrease your tolerance for that food, and then are at a greater risk of severe reaction if you try to add it back in. While elimination diets can be useful in the context of an allergy practice, we recommend avoiding trying them on your own or in other health care settings where providers might not have as much understanding and awareness of food allergies.

Nambudripad's Allergy Elimination Technique (NAET)

NAET was developed in 1983 and is purported to be a natural solution to alleviating allergies of all types and intensities. It is based on the belief that allergies are caused by an energy blockage and can be diagnosed with muscle testing. Treatment includes energy balancing and selected strategies from accupuncture/accupressure and chiropractic medicine.

There is no scientific evidence to support NAET, and it is one of the most thoroughly debunked treatment methods in this field. It is tragic that many people are still drawn to it. At least one patient has died while in "treatment" with NAET, and two licensing boards have taken regulatory action related the use of NAET

Homeopathy

The practice of homeopathy is based on the "law of similars," meaning a substance that causes a reaction can also neutralize and treat a similar reaction. It uses extremely minute doses of natural substances found in plants, animals, and minerals in remedies to strengthen and regulate the immune system. Homeopathy is found to work for about 20 percent of people with food allergies, although it is unclear what causes this beyond the placebo effect, which is a verifiable yet not-well-understood phenomenon.

In theory, homeopathy shares some similarities to food allergy immunotherapies. However, the amounts of allergens received in homeopathy are far lower than what are typically used as a starting dose of OIT. In fact, some preparations have been found to have zero molecules of active ingredient present. With OIT, the doses are gradually increased until the patient is able to eat the allergen.

Low Dose Allergy Immunotherapy (LDA)

Low dose allergy immunotherapy grew out of enzyme potentiated desensitization (EPD), which was developed in England in the 1960s. EPD injections combined very low doses of allergens with the enzyme beta-glucuronidase (normally present in the human body). EPD was administered in the United States for several years under an Investigational

Review Board study. However, when the study expired, no application was made to the FDA for Investigational New Drug (IND) status for EPD.

Low Dose Allergy Immunotherapy (LDA) is an American-made injection that includes some uniquely "New World" antigens absent in EPD, such as cottonwood, sage, mountain juniper, some evergreens, American perfumes, and avocado. LDA is believed to stimulate the regulatory arm of the immune system and dampen an allergic response. While there are plenty of anecdotes, there is scant scientific evidence that LDA works for food allergies.

Chapter 3:

Finding the Right Treatment for You

I brought my daughter to her first allergist appointment, nervous but also full of hope. This was a horrible diagnosis, but the allergist would help us fix it. Or maybe there was a mistake, and she wasn't really allergic to all those foods. I was confident that modern medicine would provide the answer.

The allergist was warm, caring, and full of information. He prescribed an EpiPen and made sure we understood how to use it. He said we shouldn't worry and that we could do this. I asked about books to read, and he gave me a few recommendations. He did not mention that only 15 percent of kids with a severe tree nut allergy ever outgrow that allergy and that there is a much greater chance of the allergy becoming more severe with age. Perhaps he thought this would be too painful for a first visit. He didn't mention that other allergists in the area offer advanced medical treatments for allergies and take kids to the point where they can free eat their allergens and live normal lives.

Even though recent scientific progress to treat food allergies has been extensive most physicians and allergists are unprepared to provide helpful information about the newly developed treatments. Even among people who are aware that treatments exist, few have up-to-date information on the variety of current options available. Allergists who do offer treatment typically only offer one type and may not be fully informed about other treatments. Every year there are more offices offering treatment, and the number of patients is rapidly expanding. Word is getting out, often spread informally through parenting communities. I have personally shared our story with hundreds of other parents and other parents who have completed treatment are similarly spreading the word.

This book is what I wished I'd had at that first allergist visit. A guide for parents, not on how to manage a severe allergy or how to hope to someday outgrow, but on how to use modern medicine to treat allergies so that their kid can live a normal life. In my opinion, treatment is easier, simpler, and far more beneficial than living life with severe food allergies.

Not all parents will choose treatment over allergen avoidance, and our society needs to continue to accommodate as best we can children who have not treated their food allergies. But all parents should at least be aware that treatments are available, and they should have good, up-to-date information on all of the options so they can make an educated choice on which treatment (if any) they would like to pursue.

Treatment Location: Private Practice vs. Clinical Trials

Food allergy treatment is generally available in two settings: private practice and clinical trials. Private practice doctors can design a treatment protocol specifically for a patient, but the depth of knowledge varies considerably from one doctor to another. Clinical trials frequently offer access to some of the best food allergy treatment minds, but protocols are not so easily tailored for a patient's specific needs. In addition, there is little to be gained personally if the child is (unknowingly to the parent) assigned to the *control group* and getting a placebo treatment.

Both treatment settings are viable options, but there are many differences. There are some things to consider when making a decision as to where to receive treatment.

- **The specific doctor who will be treating you.** Do you like the doctor? How much experience do they have with food allergy treatment and the treatment that you will be doing specifically?

Will you be primarily interacting with the doctor or with the nursing team and/or other staff? How do you feel about the support team?

- **Treatment protocol.** Would the doctor be treating just one of your allergens, multiple allergens, or *all* of your allergens? How long would treatment take, and what would be the expected end result? Would you be able to free eat your allergens, or would the treatment only allow you to tolerate a small amount of allergen?

- **Maintenance protocol.** Once treatment is completed, what would maintenance look like? How long would it last? Some doctors believe that after several years, you could drop daily maintenance requirements; others prefer that you continue maintenance requirements for life. How do you feel about your doctor's specific maintenance protocol?

- **Care after treatment.** Whichever option you select, you should know what kind of support you could get once you finish treatment. Will your doctor continue to help you if you have problems, even one to two years after completing treatment? If your initial treatment does not treat all of your allergens, would they be able to help with the additional allergens at a later date?

- **Emergency care.** What should you do in case of emergency? Will you have access to a twenty-four, seven care team, and who is the person that you will talk to in case of emergency? It may or may not be the doctor who is in charge of your treatment.

- **Travel distance.** Sometimes taking the closer option will make more sense.

- **Wait list time.** How soon would you be able to start treatment with each option? Especially in the case of younger kids, there is a real advantage to starting treatment early.

- **Possibility of placebo.** Does the clinical trial have a placebo, and, if so, would you be willing to take the chance that you might not actually get any treatment for the duration of the trial? What percentage of patients will get the placebo? Many clinical trials do offer treatment to patients who got the placebo after the trial is over, but it may mean participating in a time-consuming treatment process more than once.

- **Additional blood draws and oral food challenges.** Clinical trials generally require more consistency of blood draws and oral food challenges. Depending on your previous blood work and reaction history, a private practice doctor may not require this. On the one hand, there is some real benefit to having blood work and oral challenges confirming an allergy before you start treatment (the last thing you should be doing is completing treatment for a food that you are not actually allergic to). However, some kids are extremely adverse to blood draws and/or oral food challenges, so this may be a consideration when making your decision.

- **Interest in benefitting science and medical research.** We all benefit from the work being done in clinical trial research. Without clinical trials, we would have no good data on the outcomes of food allergy treatments. By participating in a trial, you are contributing to the advancement of science and the benefit of all patients who will be treated after you. Participating in a trial can include an educational component, with kids encouraged to learn more about the treatment that they are doing and provided with access to top scientists and researchers.

- **Cost.** Clinical trials are typically free for participants, though you will probably need to cover the cost of your travel. Private practice treatment may or may not be covered by your insurance and may be subject to deductibles, co-pays, etc.

If you are willing to do the clinical trial, the benefits to the rest of us are huge. However, some people prefer the flexibility of private practice doctors to design a treatment protocol specifically for the patient.

While private practice options are not yet universally available, their availability is growing. As an older generation of allergists retires, the younger generation is more open to the idea of trying innovative food allergy treatments. OIT is by far the most widespread treatment today and is available in most states, with over 100 allergists offering treatment. The website www.OIT101.org has a good listing of many OIT allergists across the country but does not include much information on other treatment methods besides OIT (there are some listings for SLIT). SLIT and EPIT are much more limited in availability, and FAHF-2 has only been available directly from Dr. Xiu Min Li in New York. Some satellite offices, including Dr. Jain's, are starting to offer Dr. Li's treatment through their practice.

That said, many families are willing to travel long distances to seek treatment, and some doctors offer special protocols to accommodate this. Dr Jain offers an expedited two-day rush treatment for SLIT for visitors from out of town. He also offers extended OIT appointments for people travelling for updoses. I flew across the country from California to New York to bring my kids to Dr. Li, who is associated with Mount Sinai but offers treatment in private practice. Other families relocate to be near treatment locations temporarily, typically six months to one year for OIT. Many parents consider their children's safety and health to be the single most important thing in their lives, and living with allergies is so difficult that they seek treatment, despite the significant costs in time and money.

Who Can be Treated?

Almost everyone can be treated when it is individualized for the person and their circumstances. Patients of all ages, with all allergens, and at all severities of allergies can be treated. That said, there are some general considerations that are worth keeping in mind as you read about the various treatments in upcoming chapters.

Age

Generally speaking, the younger the child, the more malleable their immune system. If you are just looking at efficacy (not risks along the way), then generally speaking, the sooner you start treatment, the better—for all treatment methods. Treatments that stimulate the regulatory side of the immune system, such as SLIT, EPIT, and FAHF-2, are more likely to take a child all the way to free eating if that child is young. Oral immunotherapy has also been shown to be most effective in younger children, but because there is a risk of severe reaction during OIT, many doctors will not begin OIT treatment until the child reaches a certain age (which ranges from two to six years old). Many doctors feel that the specific age will depend on the particular child, and they want the patient to be able to tell parents and doctors if they are having symptoms. Dr. Jain will begin SLIT and EPIT for babies and toddlers but only occasionally starts OIT before age two.

Treatments also works for older children and for adults. But for an older child with a very severe allergy, OIT may be the only option that will take the patient all the way to free eating. If you start young enough, SLIT alone may be sufficient to take a child to free eating, even for major allergens. My son is a good example of SLIT taking him to free eating for green peas. At age eleven months old, a reaction to green peas sent him to the Emergency Room for anaphylaxis. Yet by age three and a half and after completing his SLIT treatment, he was able to drink 150 mL of Ripple Milk, which is made from green peas. He also regularly drinks soy milk and eats almonds. We have reason to believe that it is possible that he could free eat other former allergens as well; however, he has become such a picky eater that we are not forcing the issue until he is older, and we are better able to communicate with him what we are trying to do.

Type of Allergies

It is generally believed that milk is one of the more challenging allergens to treat, for unclear reasons. We found that to be true with my son. He started off well, zipping along for quite some time, and he actually reached his maintenance dose of 120 mL of milk in the summer of 2016. But then unexpectedly, a few weeks later, he started reacting to his dose. We cut his dose, but he was still reacting. We cut it even further. We had to reduce his dose all the way to 30 mL before we could get him to stop reacting. We decided to hold at 30 mL for a while. Three months, to be super safe. But even after three months, my son couldn't updose beyond 30 mL. Sometimes he even reacted to his dose of 30 mL, and we were talking about possibly needing to downdose. Instead, we moved him to rush immunotherapy (more about this in the section on OIT). The rush immunotherapy seemed to help, but we were still struggling to updose him only 2.5 mL per week. Then we added back in some of the Chinese Herbs that he had been refusing (hiding them in honey on his bread). We struggled for many more months, but eventually we got him up to 60 mL by December 2016. Soon after that, he broke through the resistance zone and zoomed up to 120 mL in March 2017. Many people would have given up when faced with some of the challenges we had. It is only because of our perseverance and the amazing portfolio of treatment options used by Dr. Jain and Dr. Li that we were able to complete treatment for my son. We could easily have been part of that 20 percent that doesn't manage to complete treatment.

Severity of Allergies

Can your child tolerate a small amount of the food? Are reactions minor or severe? Unfortunately, many people (even some allergists) tell patients to assume that all food allergies should be considered life threatening.

There is good intention behind this, as it is true that even minor allergies can become more severe with time. In addition, just because a reaction has been mild in the past does not mean that it cannot be more severe in the future. Since for a long time the advice for both mild and severe allergies was avoidance, there was no real reason to distinguish between the two. However, when considering immunotherapy, treatments are different for minor and major allergens, so it is useful to make a distinction.

Dr. Jain considers "minor" allergens to be those that cause fairly mild symptoms, such as hives around the mouth or minor stomach pain. Minor allergens are also foods that can be consumed in relatively large quantities (like one-fourth of a single peanut) without reacting. "Major" allergens are allergens that result in anaphylaxis or those which cannot be tolerated even in minute amounts. High IgE levels can also be an imperfect indication of a major allergen (though there are also false positives as discussed in chapter 4). Minor allergens are much easier to treat. SLIT can take a patient all the way to free eating for a minor allergen. It is unlikely to help very much for a major allergen, though it can help get people started if they are unable to tolerate a starting dose for OIT.

When considering immunotherapy, Dr. Jain states that the most challenging patients are those with relatively narrow "therapeutic windows." The "therapeutic window" is the dose that will lead to desensitization. If you give too little of the allergen, it will do little to help desensitize the patient. If you give too much, it could cause further sensitization to the allergen. Dr. Jain says that most people have a therapeutic window that is large enough that he can work with it. But some patients have such a narrow window that it can be hard to find. These are typically the patients that are the most likely to have real setbacks with immunotherapy.

Some patients continue to have symptoms despite going incredibly slow and with tiny minute updoses. In these challenging cases, Dr. Jain sometimes uses medications to help open the therapeutic window. Xolair, Dupixent, and Dr. Li's Chinese Herbs are all treatments that can help open up the window and make the patient easier to treat with immunotherapy.

Multiple Allergens

Patients with multiple allergies, generally speaking, are harder to treat than those with fewer allergies. Protocols become more complex, and decisions need to be made about how and when to combine foods, in what order to desensitize, and what is sustainable in terms of maintenance dosing. Patients are at higher risk of anaphylactic reactions, and length of treatment could be longer than for a single allergen. That said, it can be done. I treated my daughter for thirteen severe allergies. My son was treated for an incredible forty-one allergens.

The necessity of daily (or almost daily) maintenance dosing for years is perhaps the single biggest challenge of oral immunotherapy. And the more allergens you treat, the harder it gets. For example, in my daughter's case, she needs to eat five peanuts, three hazelnuts, four pistachios, 1.5 cashews, one-half walnut, and one-half pecan. Any one of those nuts on its own would be relatively straightforward, but it is a pain to get her to eat all of them together. After her first year in maintenance, she was able to successfully switch to every-other-day dosing, which has helped a lot. Now she eats only half of the nuts every day, and we alternate the nuts that she eats (e.g., today she took peanuts, pistachios, and cashews; tomorrow she will take hazelnuts, walnuts, and pecans). It is no wonder that many people safely treat their multiple food allergies, only then to not be able to maintain the long-term dosing protocols. If you do pursue oral immunotherapy, you should be well aware of the challenge of daily maintenance dosing, especially for multiple allergens.

Both SLIT and EPIT can be easier than OIT in terms of compliance with maintenance dosing. A single bottle of SLIT drops can combine up to twenty allergens, and many (but not all!) kids don't mind doing the drops under their tongue every day. The Viaskin Patch is standardized and can only be used to treat one allergen. However, in private practice, a single customized patch can treat up to twenty allergens at the same time. The trade-off, though, is that these maintenance protocols require continued medical expenses, compared to using real food in OIT.

What Are the Desired Results?

When considering which, if any, treatment option to pursue, you should think about your long-term goals and the speed at which you hope to achieve them. Dr. Jain puts the three types of immunotherapy in order from mildest to strongest, with EPIT being the most mild, SLIT being in the middle, and OIT being the strongest. The patch will typically increase tolerance by about 3x (meaning that after treatment the patient can tolerate three times as much allergen as they could prior to treatment). So, for example, if a patient can tolerate 20mg of peanut prior to starting a patch treatment, after treatment they may be able to tolerate 60mg (still just a tiny almost-invisible speck of peanut). SLIT typically increases tolerance by about 10x. The same patient who could only tolerate 20mg would now be able to tolerate 200mg, which is about one-fourth of a single peanut. OIT can increase tolerance by 1,000x or even more. This means that the same patient could be able to tolerate 20,000mg of peanut, equivalent to about twenty-five peanuts. This is generally considered enough to allow a patient to "free eat," meaning that they can eat unlimited peanut butter sandwiches and anything else made with peanuts that they find out in the world.

That said, immunotherapy results are often surprising to all parties involved. FAHF-2 is unlikely to take patients all the way to free eating for the most severe allergens, though it has worked for some patients. In the case of my daughter, Dr. Li told us it was unlikely that FAHF-2 would take her all the way to free eating. We ended up combining FAHF-2 with SLIT, and to the surprise and delight of both Dr. Jain and Dr. Li, this did take her all the way to free eating for her fish allergy (with IgE>100).

Some treatments are faster than others. Dr. Jain's SLIT treatment is one of the fastest available, typically taking about one month if updosing goes smoothly. Patch treatment can also be very fast, depending on the protocol. Oral immunotherapy is the next fastest, averaging six months to a year of regular visits in order to reach maintenance dose. For some patients, they may be able to reach maintenance as quickly as three months but for others it can take over a year. It should be noted, however, that building up to maintenance dose is only one phase of the treatment and this is followed by a "long tail" of maintenance requirements. Your child will be protected and able to eat their allergens; however, they will be required to eat them regularly (or continue SLIT dosing) for at least a few more years before possibly reaching sustained tolerance. SLIT using the La Crosse method and FAHF-2 typically all require years worth of treatment before oral challenges are attempted.

Willingness to Follow Challenging Protocols

Protocols are not easy. While they vary from one treatment method to another, you are probably looking at several years of hard work if you want to treat a severe food allergy. Treating multiple severe allergies is even harder. None of the food allergy treatments provide an easy or quick fix. Real world factors such as number of adults at home, work flexibility, distance to travel for treatment, other children/childcare responsibilities, and extracurricular activities (to name just a few), can and will impact willingness to follow a treatment protocol. So too will risk tolerance and ability to manage anxiety, both for parents and children.

In terms of the active treatment phase, it is probably safe to say that EPIT and SLIT are the easiest protocols to follow, with OIT being in the middle (harder for multiple allergens) and FAHF-2 being the most challenging. OIT, SLIT, and sometimes EPIT require an updosing phase, with increases that are typically done in the doctor's office. These require frequent visits to the doctor's office, usually every one to two weeks. Appointments often occur during school hours, leading to missed classroom time. And, of course, that also means missed work time for parents. Protocols may involve eating your allergen every day, taking daily drops, changing your patch every one to three days, or taking large numbers of pills.

Once you reach the maintenance phase, protocols become more straightforward. Drops under the tongue once a day for SLIT (or three times a day with the La Crosse Protocol). Patch protocol typically requires changing the patch every one to three days. OIT maintenance requires eating a certain amount of food daily (or, eventually, a few times a week).

The amount that you need to eat varies by patient, by doctor, and by allergen. Using peanuts as an example, some allergists like Dr. Jain generally stop at five peanuts but allow their patients to increase to "free eating" if they so wish by increasing the amount eaten at home (outside of dosing). One doctor takes his patients all the way to where they eat sixty peanuts a day for a little while before then reducing the amount, though sometimes requiring sixty peanuts once a week after that. It is worth looking into the specific protocol of the allergist you are considering treatment with and adding up all the foods that will require daily dosing.

Many babies and young toddlers can be treated without their even knowing what is going on. Other babies and toddlers may be challenging to treat, since they are not old enough even to be bribed into consenting to treatment. As a baby, my son was happy to take a nasty concoction of herbs mixed with Zyrtec and Splenda and was willing to take herbal baths and get covered in green creams several times a day. He was also eager to drink his milk every day (it was the only time we would let him drink from a bottle) and take sweet drops under his tongue once a day. Just before he turned three years old, he got much more stubborn. He started refusing the nasty concoction of herbs and protesting the baths and creams. He is still happy to drink his milk twice a day and willing to put up with the drops under his tongue.

Once your child is around age four or five, you really need the child to be on board for treatment. Especially for OIT and FAHF-2, where treatment protocols are the most challenging. Even if a child starts out interested in pursuing treatment, the challenge of daily protocols may cause them to change their minds. Many patients undergoing OIT and FAHF-2 have hidden their doses at one time or another (more about that later). So if you have an older child, it is really important that they see the benefit before you begin treatment.

Not all kids understand the benefit of food allergy treatment. As parents, we can go so far out of our way to make their lives "normal" that they may not see the downside of having a food allergy. Some parents, especially of young teens, have found that they need to have their child take control of the challenging aspects of managing their allergy in order to understand the benefits of treatment. When they always magically have their own safe meals and treats, provided by a parent, they may not see why things need to change.

Cost

At the time of writing, the cost of treatment varies widely from one practitioner to another. Insurance coverage also varies considerably. The cost of treatments is based on the total number of updoses. Generally speaking, the fewer updoses, the cheaper the treatment. If the patient starts at a higher dose, the cost will be lower. If the patient reaches any "resistance points" during treatment and has to slow down and/or the doctor has to create intermediary steps between doses, then the cost will be more. It is, therefore, very challenging to estimate the total cost prior to starting treatment. Some doctors also offer "rush immunotherapy," meaning that they updose more than once in a single visit. An individual appointment will be longer and potentially more expensive, though fewer appointments will be needed.

Once you reach the maintenance stage, costs will change. OIT is typically only expensive in the treatment phase, as real food is generally used for maintenance dosing. In contrast, SLIT and EPIT will require either switching to real food (which may require OIT or a modified OIT protocol done at home), or maintenance doses that are prepared by the doctor and are considerably more expensive than regular food from the supermarket.

While I hesitate to include any pricing information, since it will immediately be out of date as soon as the book is published, some current price range for treatments are set out below:

- **Oral Immunotherapy (OIT):** $200–$2,000 per appointment during the updosing phase. Just the cost of food once you reach maintenance (unless you are staying on the Aimmune peanut pill).

- **Sublingual Immunotherapy (SLIT):** $100–$1,000 per appointment during the updosing phase; $70–200 per bottle (holding up to twenty allergens) per month once you reach maintenance (unless you switch to regular food).

- **Epicutaneous Immunotherapy (EPIT/Patch):** $100–$200 per appointment during the updosing phase; $100 per month once you reach maintenance (unless you switch to regular food).

- **FAHF-2:** Typically between $300 and $800 per month, depending on the protocol. Treatment lasts two to four years.

I recommend you contact the providers you are considering to find out the likely costs. Most doctors strongly advise you contact them directly instead of contacting your health insurance company, who may be unfamiliar with the billing codes used and may tell you that they do not cover treatment. Quite a few families in treatment (our family included) change health insurance plans so that they get the best possible coverage for the year(s) in which they are planning to do food allergy treatment.

Many doctors accept health insurance for OIT, SLIT, and EPIT and bill office visits to insurance. There may be an additional noncovered charge for the immunotherapy doses. I have not yet heard of any cases of insurance covering the cost of FAHF-2, although health-spending accounts can be used to cover the cost of the herbs if there is a letter of medical necessity.

Chapter 4:

Preparing for Treatment

There are a number of things you can do prior to starting food allergy treatment that will make your journey easier and faster. These include confirming which allergies are true allergies requiring treatment, treating environmental allergies, and getting eczema and asthma under control. These preparations can be done with your local allergist or with your treatment allergist, depending on your individual situation.

Allergy Testing

One of the first things that patients typically do after encountering problems with a food is allergy testing through blood work and/or skin prick tests. Unfortunately, food allergy testing is not straightforward and requires the help of an experienced allergist to administer and interpret tests. The high rate of false positives in blood and skin tests can cause undue stress and anxiety. They are the reason that many allergists prefer not to even test unless there is a history of reaction or other good reason to suspect an allergy. Combining blood tests and skin tests with clinical history gives the most comprehensive information.

Before I go more into the widely accepted and used methods for diagnosing food allergies, I would like to mention a handful of alternative testing methods you might run into. None of these are scientifically proven or standardized. Tests to avoid include the following: applied kinesiology (muscle testing), electrodermal testing, NAET or Nambrudipad's Allergy Elimination Technique, IgG testing, hair analysis, and pulse testing.

Blood Tests

Bloodwork measures the level of immunoglobulin E (IgE), antibodies that are responsible for triggering an allergic reaction. It is common to look at both total serum IgE levels, as well as food-specific IgE. In general, the higher the food-specific IgE level, the more likely it is that the person has a true allergy. A higher number does not necessarily indicate how severe your allergy is or how likely you are to have an anaphylactic response. According to FARE, blood tests show false positives 50 to 60 percent of the time. This means that more than half of the time that blood tests suggest an allergy, you are not actually allergic! False negatives are less common but do still happen. My son tested positive for some legumes but not for all of them, so he did several food challenges for foods that we thought he would be able to tolerate. However, on his second dose of green beans (with IgE<0.35, the lowest possible amount), he had an anaphylactic reaction.

Cutting-edge treatment allergists may use newer blood tests involving component-resolved diagnostics for certain foods. These tests provide a more nuanced look at allergies by identifying IgE levels specific to different proteins within a single food. This information has important implications in understanding the severity and risk of a given allergy, as well as potential for desensitization. For example, certain proteins in peanut are associated with a high risk of anaphylaxis, while another protein is associated with lower risk of systemic reaction and a greater likelihood of long-term tolerance. In the hands of an experienced treatment allergist, this information can help guide treatment planning and choices.

Some doctors also test for biomarkers, trying to better understand specific allergens. However, it is worth noting that, while the use of biomarkers may provide useful information for scientists, they currently do not have any clinical or practical utility and are not recommended for diagnosing or treating food allergies. All of the treatment methods and tests described in this book have been detailed in the scientific and peer-reviewed literature, meaning that they have met some minimum standard of scrutiny by their peers. The use of biomarkers has so far not shown sufficient reliability to be incorporated in the protocols for management of food allergies.

Skin Prick Tests

Skin prick tests involve placing a drop of the allergen being tested on your back or arm. The skin is then pricked or scratched to allow a tiny amount to enter into the body. Positive results are indicated by a wheal (a raised white bump surround by red itchy skin). In general, the larger the wheal, the more likely you are to have a true allergy. Skin tests also have a high false-positive rate, estimated to be more than 50 percent. False negatives are rare, and it is unlikely that there is an allergy if the skin test is negative.

Even with the risk of false positives and negatives, food allergy testing is usually done prior to starting treatment. We know that results change over time and that many children will outgrow allergies over time. Rather than relying on outdated results, your doctor will want current testing. After all, the last thing anyone wants is to undergo a challenging treatment protocol for a nonexistent allergy. Based on blood and skin test results, an oral challenge with suspected foods is likely the next step.

Oral Food Challenges

Oral food challenges are the gold standard for food allergy diagnosis, as they are close to 100 percent accurate. If you have any doubts, then the best way to determine whether your child is truly allergic is with an oral challenge. Remember, despite positive blood and/or skin test results, if your child can eat a food with no symptoms, they are not allergic.

In addition to helping diagnose allergies, oral challenges yield important information about the amount of allergen that can be tolerated. For decades, allergists have generally taken a "pass/fail" approach to food allergies. This means that, if you fail an oral food challenge at the final dose, you are told to avoid the food entirely. Recent research has suggested that keeping small amounts of allergens in your diet may actually help push the patient into "outgrowing" the allergy. While this is still an area where additional study is needed, it is worth considering that strict avoidance may not always be the best advice. In many cases, these "almost passes" may be treated at home and may not require formal medical treatment.

Dr. Jain uses a different approach to oral food challenges, which include not only "pass/fail" options but also what he calls an "almost pass." An almost pass is when a person reacts to the food during the challenge, but either the reaction is not severe or it is to a relatively high dose. After an almost pass, the patient is encouraged to eat the food regularly, but only in amounts smaller than the final amount tolerated at the oral challenge. This will help build tolerance for that food, which can be then challenged again at a later date.

My daughter almost passed her challenge to macadamia nuts. She was able to tolerate one-half of a macadamia nut just fine but had a stomachache when she ate one full nut. Dr. Jain encouraged us to feed her one-half of a nut regularly at home to increase her tolerance. He said that there was no need to treat this allergy with oral immunotherapy; we could just increase her tolerance at home. In contrast, at age three, Layla started complaining that walnuts (which she had been eating previously) made her mouth hurt. We consulted her previous allergist, who told us to completely remove walnuts from her diet to be "on the safe side." In the coming years, we continued to avoid walnuts, and she became much more severely allergic to them. Had I gone back in time, I would have kept walnuts in her diet but in smaller portions. Perhaps if she had regularly kept eating just one-fourth of a walnut every day, we could have avoided the need for oral immunotherapy. I wonder how many of the foods that our kids are strictly avoiding could (and should!) actually be incorporated into their diets, to help push them in the direction of "outgrowing" the allergy. These conversations and decisions should only be made under the guidance of a knowledgeable allergist.

If you do decide to pursue immunotherapy, any knowledge that you have about the amount of allergen that can be safely tolerated will help you determine the best treatment for you. As an example, prior to seeking treatment with Dr. Jain, my son did a baked milk challenge with his previous allergist. He failed the challenge when he ate one-eighth of a small cupcake with milk in it (that's a crumb about the size of a thumbnail). Our allergist gave us no advice other than that it was "a disappointing result." A few months later, we sought treatment with Dr. Jain, and I told him about the challenge. He was very pleased that I was able to provide the information that my son could eat one-sixteenth of a cupcake (a tiny crumb) with no reaction, and he was able to suggest that we start baked milk OIT at the dose of one-sixteenth of a cupcake.

As you can see, oral food challenges are very helpful, but they do have some downsides. To begin with, they are time consuming and must be done one at a time for each potential allergen. Each oral food challenge typically takes about four hours. In cases where there is no reason to suspect a serious food allergy, they can be done at home. If there is good reason to suspect a serious allergy, though, they typically must be done at an allergist's office. Another big downside to oral food challenges is the risk of a severe reaction. If you suspect that your child is allergic to a food, then it can be scary to feed that food to your child and wait to see if they react. The fact that they may react with anaphylaxis can make the challenge even more frightening

However, if you can manage it, I personally think that there is a real benefit to having a child experience anaphylaxis in a medical setting. You and your child can see what anaphylaxis is like and how easily it can be treated with epinephrine. Most parents have deep anxiety about using an epinephrine autoinjector. Having the parent inject the child in the doctor's office, with medical supervision, is an incredible opportunity to face this fear in a safe environment.

The first time I used epinephrine, I was at home and terrified. Even though her reaction didn't seem life-threatening (mild wheezing and hives), what if I did it wrong? I was tempted to call 911 or just administer Benadryl and hope for the best. But thankfully, our allergist had told me that this sort of fear is normal and that the best thing I could do was get over my fear by using epinephrine, even if I wasn't totally sure it was necessary. And so with my heart beating in my ears, I held down my three-year-old daughter and gave her a shot in the leg. She immediately started breathing easier, and I felt like a hero. What a boost to my confidence and my ability to manage my kids' allergies! The second time I used epinephrine was when my eleven-month-old son had an allergic reaction at daycare. By the time I got there, he had hives all over his body and couldn't breathe properly. He had never been prescribed an EpiPen, but I had one in my purse for his sister. As soon as I saw him, I immediately knew what to do and didn't hesitate. I grabbed the EpiPen, grabbed my son, and injected him in the leg. He immediately felt better and could breathe again.

Giving epinephrine can be very scary, which is why it is so important to practice doing it. Getting over the hurdle of doing it for the first time creates a certain amount of confidence, which makes administering the drug a second time, in unforeseen circumstances, easier to do. I now see oral food challenges as an opportunity for other caregivers to get over their fear of using epinephrine. My husband administered epinephrine for the first time ever during our son's failed green bean challenge. He tells me that he now feels better prepared to do it if it is ever needed in the outside world. As my daughter got older, I was planning to help her learn to self-administer during oral food challenges. She never got the chance, since she passed her last four food challenges following treatment. But had she failed any one of them, it would have been an incredible opportunity for her to start to take charge of her own treatment. I had also been planning on inviting the kids' grandparents and our babysitter to oral food challenges so that they could really learn how to administer epinephrine.

A note about the accuracy of oral food challenges: There are cases of people passing a food challenge but then reacting to a food days or weeks later. Generally speaking, this can happen when someone is able to tolerate a certain amount of a food but is technically still allergic and has developed a tolerance similar to what is gained through immunotherapy. Then if they are sick, tired, or have hormonal changes, they may be more susceptible to reacting to the food. In these cases, an experienced oral immunotherapy allergist can help you find the dose of the food that your child is able to tolerate safely at home, and you may want to respect some of the same limitations as those in immunotherapy treatment (e.g., lower the dose if sick, tired, etc.).

New allergies can also develop following an illness or a course of antibiotics. My son had been eating green peas semiregularly before he had a bad cold and subsequently had his first anaphylactic reaction to peas. This can be terrifying. It's also a good reason to always carry your epinephrine auto-injector, even if you're not planning on feeding your child anything that you know they are allergic to.

Treating Environmental Allergies

Before beginning food allergy treatment, it may make sense to test for and treat environmental allergies (e.g., pollen, dust, pets, etc.). You may wish to do a full panel of environmental allergy tests, as there may be some unknown environmental allergies that are causing issues, and they can all be treated together. Most food allergic children also have environmental allergies, although some parents are unaware of these allergies or deem them less important since they are not life-threatening. Yet reactions to environmental allergens are easily confused with reactions to foods, and treating environmental allergies can reduce sensitivities to foods. Those are two good reasons to treat environmental allergies prior to starting treatment for food allergies.

The most effective way of treating environmental allergies is typically with allergy shots, which are readily available in much of the world. However, allergy shots do require a long-term commitment and frequent visits to the allergist's office. If you are looking for something a bit more flexible, you could also consider SLIT. You do not need to see an allergist on a regular basis, and it might be more appealing to patients who have issues with shots. However, you do typically need to take the drops every day at home, so compliance is sometimes not as good as for allergy shots.

Oral Allergy Syndrome (OAS) can be dramatically improved by treating the underlying environmental allergies that cause OAS (e.g., birch pollen allergy is a common one). Once this is done, many patients find that their allergic symptoms to foods disappear. This works in approximately 60 to 80 percent of cases. For example, my tongue used to hurt if I ate walnuts. It was a small nuisance, and I occasionally continued to eat walnuts despite the discomfort. Dr. Jain told me that it was probably OAS and that it would be relatively easy to treat the allergy. I was planning to treat my environmental allergies anyway, and sure enough, SLIT did the trick. I can now eat walnuts without any pain in my mouth.

If treating your environmental allergies doesn't provide enough relief, then you can treat your OAS directly with food sublingual (SLIT) immunotherapy. Not that many allergists in the United States currently offer this treatment method, but it is increasingly becoming available, so it's worth asking around your local area. Treatment can take as little as a few days if you are willing to travel to some of the innovators (like Dr. Jain), though you will need to stay on "maintenance" drops of your allergens for a few years. Sadly, the drops are generally not covered by health insurance, so they are usually a more expensive option for long-term maintenance than allergy shots.

Controlling Asthma and Eczema

Asthma must be under control before you can begin food allergy immunotherapy treatments. You may already be familiar with conventional medications for controlling asthma, which can be prescribed by your doctor. These medications (including steroids) are generally safe and effective, though they can have some negative side effects. Xolair, and other biologics such as Dupixent, are incredible drugs that are given as a shot and can make a dramatic difference in asthma symptoms. But as with steroids, these medications provide relief, not a longer-term cure.

Most doctors talk about controlling the symptoms of asthma, not treating the underlying condition. Treatments that address the underlying causes of asthma can greatly reduce the need for conventional medications.

Two methods of doing this are treating environmental allergies with SLIT or allergy shots as well as the Chinese herbal Anti-Asthma Simplified Herbal Medicine Intervention (ASHMI).

Environmental allergies can be treated, either via allergy shots or SLIT, and many people find that treating these environmental allergies provides enormous asthma relief and reduces the need for conventional medications. You can work with an allergist to help identify and treat your environmental allergies. ASHMI comes out of Mt. Sinai in New York (a well-established scientific research hospital) and has demonstrated the ability to treat asthma and seems to be as effective as controller medications. It is available to the public through Dr. Li's private practice.

My kids both suffer from asthma. Both of them used to be on regular nebulizer treatments throughout the winter, with semiregular use during the rest of the year. Before we started treatment, my daughter's asthma was not well controlled, and she was using her rescue medication more than twice a week. My son's asthma was even worse than his sister's, and he was using the nebulizer twice a day. We have seen real improvements since having the kids go through SLIT for environmental allergies and ASHMI. We still keep my daughter (now eleven) on one of her controller medications (Singulair), but she only uses the second (Flovent) when she has a cold or after an asthma flare. Her symptoms are far better than they were a few years ago. My son, now seven, is completely off all asthma medications. We generally still put him on a controller medication when he gets a cold as a preventative measure, but he has only used his nebulizer once in the past year.

Treating asthma helps make treating food allergies safer and smoother, but it is also an incredible achievement just in itself. Far more kids die every year from asthma than from food allergies. Before you treat your kid's food allergies, it's worth seriously thinking about how you might treat the underlying allergies that are causing asthma.

Table 1: Comparison of Immunotherapy Treatments

Picking the right treatment for you

	OIT	SLIT	Patch	FAHF-2
Effectiveness	Can increase tolerance by 1,000x or more.	Typically increases tolerance by about 10x.	Typically increases tolerance by about 3x.	Reduces the total allergenic load; may not take patient to free eating for severe allergies.
Severity of the allergy	OIT is ideal for the most severe allergies. It is burdensome for minor allergies.	May provide freedom from cross contamination for severe allergies, free eating for minor allergies.	May provide freedom from cross contamination for severe allergies, free eating for minor allergies.	Helps for all levels of severity. May not take patient to free eating for severe allergies.
Age of patient	Works well on children and adults of all ages, but because of risks involved many start at age 2-6.	Is most effective on younger kids (even babies and toddlers), but can treat patients of any age.	Is most effective on younger kids, but can treat patients of any age.	Is most effective on younger kids (even babies and toddlers), but can treat patients of any age.
Protocol ease	Maintenance protocols are challenging for most, especially for multiple allergens.	Protocols are relatively easy for most people.	Protocols are relatively easy for most people.	Protocols are extremely challenging for most people.
Number of allergens	Gets more challenging the more allergens are treated.	Easy - can treat up to 20 allergens in a single vial.	Custom patches can treat up to 20 allergens. Pharmaceutical patches are for a single allergen.	Single protocol treats all allergens at the same time.
Speed of treatment	Typically 4-12 months to treat, 3+ years of maintenance.	Typically 1-2 months to treat, 3+ years of maintenance (or transition to OIT).	Typically 1-6 months to treat, 3+ years of maintenance (or transition to SLIT/OIT).	Typically 2-4 years of treatment, no maintenance requirements.

Part II
Evidence Based Treatments

Chapter 5:

Oral Immunotherapy

Oral immunotherapy (OIT) is probably the most widespread treatment for food allergies. Any food allergy can be treated with OIT, and it can work for even the most severe (anaphylactic) allergies. It works by gradually increasing tolerance for a food, starting with minuscule amounts. Treatment typically takes four to six months or more, and you will have to continue to eat your allergens regularly for at least a few years after finishing treatment. If you have a severe allergy and your goal is to be able to eat as much of your allergen as you wish, OIT is a great treatment option.

There are some downsides of OIT to consider. Minor reactions during treatment are common, and about 10 to 20 percent of patients have severe reactions. For many patients this is a major barrier to treatment with OIT. If you are treating multiple allergies, continuing to eat all of those foods regularly for years can be burdensome. Even with creative dosing ideas and schedules, the long-tail of maintenance is challenging. Finally, some people are concerned that OIT is not FDA approved. As discussed previously, OIT as it is currently practiced uses regular food for treatment and, therefore, does not fall under the auspices of the FDA, as there is no medication to evaluate. Some of these concerns may be alleviated by the January 2020 approval of Aimmune's "peanut pill" called Palforzia, discussed in more depth in chapter 6. This approval validates the theory and protocols of oral immunotherapy in use today by reputable allergists. And while Palforzia is now officially approved for treatment of peanut allergy, private practice allergists are able to customize similar treatments for virtually any food allergy.

OIT treatments vary depending on the provider, the patient, and the allergen being treated. In this section I will discuss some of the basic tenements of *most* OIT protocols. However, it is important to note that, while these protocols hold for the majority of OIT providers, they do not hold for all of them. And even providers who follow this process for most of their OIT patients will vary it depending on the specific circumstances of a patient. Special considerations in OIT treatment will be discussed in chapter 6.

Preparing for OIT

Prior to starting OIT, you will have a consultation with your treatment allergist and may do additional tests (e.g., skin tests, blood tests, oral challenges). The more informed you are about the OIT process, the better you can help your allergist understand what may or may not work for you and your family. For example, you may know that it will be impractical for you to continue with maintenance protocols for more than four or five foods simultaneously because of the amount of food involved. This information will help you and your allergist decide which foods should be treated with oral immunotherapy and which may be better off with another treatment method. Similarly, thinking about how much food you would like to be able to eat is another important factor. Are you looking for "free eating," or would you prefer "safe from cross contamination"?

It is also worth considering the form that your maintenance dose will take. My experience and those of my friends is that kids tend to have a much harder time with nut and egg maintenance than with milk or wheat. After completing multi-nut OIT with my daughter, I could not even contemplate fish OIT, where she would have to eat fish every day (or perhaps *almost* every day). If you know your goals and how much dosing you think you can handle in maintenance, you will be in a good position to work with your allergist to develop a treatment plan that is specific for your needs and works for your family. You may now be ready to schedule your appointment for OIT Day 1!

OIT Treatment Phase

Day 1 of OIT

Prior to your arrival for your first OIT appointment, your allergist or another team member will precisely calculate and measure the starting dose. The starting dose will vary, depending on the doctor and the allergen, but it is typically on the order of 0.1mg of allergen; that's about the same weight as one-sixth of a grain of salt. Some allergists start as low as 0.01mg of allergen. That is a *truly* tiny speck of allergen, one-sixtieth of a grain of salt. In some cases (for example if you failed an oral challenge prior to starting OIT), your allergist may already know that you can tolerate a larger amount of allergen. For instance, they might know that your child could tolerate 0.1 grams, because that is the dose that they passed, before failing at the next stage of the oral challenge. In those cases, the starting dose may be closer to the last dose successfully challenged (e.g., 0.1 grams).

When you arrive at the allergist's office, you will be shown into a room where you can expect to spend the next one to eight hours. The amount of time you will spend in the office will vary on the protocol; some allergists do only a single dose on Day 1, many of them do multiple doses. You should know how long your appointment is expected to last, though it will probably be shorter if your child has a reaction to one of the doses.

Soon after you arrive, a nurse or other team member will arrive to check vitals, ask about any recent illnesses, and make sure that you are ready to go. Assuming that you and your child are ready, the team member will then prepare the dose. You may have been asked to bring your own "mixer" or "medium" for the dose; the most common is applesauce, though some parents prefer pudding, yogurt, or other soft foods. I'm going to assume it is applesauce for the sake of simplicity. A few minutes later, the team member will return with a spoonful of applesauce with the dose mixed in. Your child will eat the dose and take a sip of water or juice to wash it down. You will then wait twenty to thirty minutes to make sure there is no reaction. It's good to keep a close eye on your child during this waiting period, as you are expected to report any symptoms, like hives, that kids may not notice.

The nurse will come back after the waiting period to check on your child and take vitals again. Assuming that everything looks good, the nurse will then bring the next dose, perhaps 0.2mg of allergen, and you will repeat the process of waiting and checking vitals. If there is still no reaction, then the patient may increase to 0.4mg, and then 0.6mg. Some doctors do as many as eight to ten updoses on the first day of treatment. Dr. Jain typically stops after four updoses, even if there are no symptoms.

Common minor reactions include stomachaches, hives, flushing, or vomiting. If there is a minor reaction on Day 1, then the doctor and/or the nursing team will evaluate whether the reaction was minor enough that the patient should stop, try again at the same dose (there's a better chance that there will be no reaction the second time around), or try a smaller increase than the previous does that was tolerated. Many factors are included in this evaluation, including the patient's allergic history, their temperament, and even nap schedules for younger kids (patients are more likely to have an allergic reaction if they are tired). Severe reactions (e.g., anaphylaxis) on Day 1 are rare but they do happen. If that occurs, then the allergist will typically administer epinephrine, stop treatment, and either dramatically reduce the starting dose (to be given on a different day) or switch to another treatment method like SLIT to increase the starting tolerance before restarting OIT.

Whatever highest dose your child reaches on Day 1, that will then be their "at home" dose for the next week or two. Some allergists, like Dr. Jain, give the second-to-last dose as the "at home" dose because it reduces the risk of a reaction at home. So, for example, if a patient reaches 0.6mg allergen on Day 1 (as my daughter did), then she will take at home just 0.4mg of the allergen. Depending on the food being treated and the doctor's protocol, the patient will then need to take this dose once or twice a day until they come back into the allergist's office for the next updose.

Tips and Tricks for Day 1

There is a lot that you can do to help ensure a smooth Day 1. You may be extremely nervous. Depending on your child's age, he or she may be equally nervous. It may be helpful to connect with other families who have been through treatment. Your doctor may be able to suggest some names, and Facebook is an incredible resource for connecting with other families. There are many private OIT groups online and even private groups just for kids to connect with other kids.

Another thing that helps with Day 1 is entertainment. Especially if you're going to be in the office for four to eight hours, you're going to need a lot of things to do while you wait. If all goes well and there are no allergic reactions, OIT visits will be long and boring. Many patients bring a rolling suitcase worth of things for the day, including books, games, toys, snacks and possibly lunch (for the kids *and* the adults), and some sort of digital entertainment (iPad, Kindle, DVD player, etc.). On my initial visit, I didn't realize how much entertainment would be needed and naively brought almost nothing. But by my second visit, I was the one rolling in a suitcase full of entertainment, with other families commenting that they wish they had thought of that. Personally, I like to begin the day with games and books and save the iPad and digital media for the second half of the visit, when we all start going a bit crazy. I found that it was easy to switch from classical entertainment to electronic entertainment, but it was much harder for my kids to switch from electronic entertainment to books and physical games. Of course, you are likely to know what will work best for your own kids.

Another trick I used was wrapping small presents for each dose. I would stock up on small and inexpensive "gifts," such as stickers, crayons, coloring books, and card games, and give my kids a wrapped "gift" after each updose. This certainly helped pass the time. Sidewalk chalk is another excellent option for allergist offices if the patient has the option of going outside between doses.

It's also lovely to connect with other families who are in treatment. Some offices have a communal space with a few toys where you can go between doses and checks. This is a favorite spot for many kids, who prefer to play with other kids, and also for parents, who can connect with one another. Even in offices where each patient is in their own room with no formal communal space, I found it easy to connect with other families. Occasionally I would post a note on our doctor-specific Facebook group that I was in room 4 if anyone wanted to come by and say hello, and people would. It was a wonderful way to meet and connect with other families in treatment, share stories, and support one another. Unfortunately with COVID-19, communal space is no longer practical, but social media remains a vital means of connecting with other families undergoing similar experiences.

Day 1 is exhausting for kids, and it is exhausting for most parents too. Be sure to bring some treats for yourself, as well as for your kids. If you can tag-team with a coparent, let them know that Day 1 will wipe you out and have them take the kids the instant you get home. I took both my kids to their Day 1 appointments (not on the same day), and in both cases, my husband took the kids the second we got home, and I got a much-needed break.

Some families with multiple kids needing treatment do take their kids to appointments at the same time. Most parents I know feel that this is more than twice as hard as an OIT appointment with just one kid, but at the same time the dramatic reduction in time off work required, travel time, and total appointment time may make it worth it.

You did it—you are officially on the path to treating your kid's allergies. Congratulations on a successful Day 1!

At Home Dosing

After starting OIT, you will need to dose at home until it is time to go back to the allergist's office for the next updose. Your allergist will probably send you home with a bunch of premeasured doses, which will last you until your next appointment. Every day (and sometimes twice a day), you will mix your dose with applesauce (or whatever food you choose) and give it to your child. Dosing at home requires vigilance on the part of the patient or parent as well as a willingness to accept a certain degree of risk. If you aren't comfortable with this risk, then you might want to consider a different treatment option. While in theory there should be no reactions at home, that doesn't mean that there aren't. Most people I know who have completed OIT have had at least one minor reaction at home. Reactions happen more often if your child gets sick, if he or she is overly active, or if there are any environmental changes. Beware of vacations and weekend trips! My daughter reacted to doses that had previously been just fine when we were travelling. You should already have an EpiPen (or equivalent) and know how to use it.

Your allergist will probably ask you to respect a "rest period" before and after your child doses at home. This is because exercise can increase the likelihood of the dose causing an allergic reaction. The rest period typically extends from an hour before the dose, to two hours after the dose is taken. There is also an "observation period" for one hour after the dose, during which time you should keep an eye on your child, checking for signs of a mild allergic reaction. I find TV time and car time are ideal for rest periods. There's nothing quite like having your kid become a sedentary zombie in front of the TV or having them physically restrained by seat belts, to ensure that they are "resting." For the littlest kids (ages three and under), it may be next to impossible to enforce a rest period. My son could not sit still during OIT. Even while watching TV, he frequently got up and ran around the house before going back to finish watching his program. If we lock him into his high-chair for too long, he throws a tantrum (which can also provoke an allergic reaction). We eventually gave up and accepted that he just wasn't going to be able to have a proper rest period. A good allergist will work with you—and within the limits of what is and what isn't possible for your family.

In the morning, a dose may be given soon after you wake up (say, 7:00 a.m.), though ideally doses shouldn't be given on an empty stomach. We usually just give my kids something small before they take their doses; a full breakfast takes too long, and we need to dose early to have sufficient time for the observation period before we leave for school and work. The observation period is over when we leave (8:00 a.m.), and the rest period extends into the first hour of school (9:00 a.m.), during which time our kids are typically engaged in (relatively) calm morning welcoming activities. If your child has PE for their first class in the morning, you may need to ask for special accommodations or dose earlier in the morning.

In the evening, we try to have our kids stop afterschool sports activities by 6:00 p.m. so that they can take their dose at 7:00 p.m. (right after dinner) and be observed until 8:00 p.m. OIT can be challenging to manage for kids who are very active on sports teams. My daughter was doing serious gymnastics while in OIT, and we had to rearrange her practice schedule to make dosing work.

If your kid becomes sick, then there is an increased risk that there could be an allergic reaction to the at-home dose. For this reason, you will probably be advised to call the allergist if there is any sign that the patient is ill. Minor colds are less of a problem, but a fever or stomach bug can greatly increase the chance of a reaction. Your allergist will probably ask you to decrease your at-home dose for a few days, until your child has fully recovered from the illness. In fact, they probably gave you a few lower doses to take home with you during your in-office appointment just so that you would be ready in case of illness.

After at least a week of home dosing, and assuming there have been no reactions at home, you are now ready for your next updose appointment.

Updosing Visits

After the first visit, you will continue to come to the allergist's office every week or two for an "updose." Some allergists do a single updose in the office every week, in which case you may only be at the allergist's office for a bit over an hour. Others, like Dr. Jain, continue with multiple updoses over the course of half a day. I brought my rolling suitcase into every updose appointment. Even so, my kids quickly decided that they would rather play with *other* kids' toys. Thankfully, we quickly made friends with other families who had similar updosing schedules and had the opportunity to share and exchange toys as well as our experiences.

After each updose appointment, if your kid can tolerate the new increased dose, then that is the new amount that you will take home.

Similar to Day 1, if your child has any sort of reaction, then you will either hold at the previous dose, updose less than otherwise, or possibly even decrease to a lower dose. The amount of dose increase each visit varies a lot, but as a good rule of thumb, if there are no symptoms, you might expect your child to roughly double the amount of allergen he or she can tolerate every appointment. If there are zero symptoms along the way, then your child could get through the updosing phase in as little as four months.

My daughter did this for buckwheat, finishing updosing in four months with only a few extremely minor symptoms along the way. This was despite the fact that on paper (and in our experience), her allergy to buckwheat was far more severe than her allergy to peanuts and tree nuts. Multiple nuts took her seven months to complete, including about a month "off" during the winter holidays.

Milk OIT is often more challenging than other foods and also takes longer. Because of some of the specific challenges surrounding desensitization of milk, eggs, fish, and shellfish, the next chapter covers these foods in more detail. Milk is generally considered one of the toughest allergies to treat. It took my son about eighteen months to complete the updosing phase of milk OIT, which is longer than average. The average for milk OIT is probably about six to twelve months.

Kids and parents typically have to take time off school and work for allergist appointments during OIT. If the allergist doing the treatment is local, you may only need to take off half a day from school and work, and this could be done every other week or less frequently if needed. Some parents try to schedule accelerated OIT for their kids over the summer with weekly updoses, and do every other week updoses during the rest of the year. Most schools are willing to accommodate OIT.

All public schools are required to accommodate updosing appointments if you include OIT as part of your 504 plan (a plan that most severely allergic kids in public schools have in place to manage their allergy). Because missing school and work can be challenging, OIT can be easier for younger kids and families where at least one parent has a flexible schedule. But OIT is also commonly done by teenagers and families with two working parents. Many families choose to make sacrifices so that it will work.

My husband and I would alternate taking the kids to their OIT appointments. I think it can be helpful to share responsibility with your partner if you can, as it allows both of you to learn more about the process and what to look for in case of reaction. My husband is now better than I am at spotting the minor symptoms of bumpy skin and redness around my son's mouth when he's having a mild allergic reaction.

Graduation Day

The final dose that a patient needs to reach in order to "graduate" OIT varies from one doctor to another, but it is typically between four and eight grams of the food (for peanuts, that is typically between five and ten peanuts). Once the final dose is reached, the patient typically holds at that dose for at least a month, and then Dr. Jain allows patients to begin gradually introducing that food into their diet. Most allergists ask that their patients pass a "super challenge" (for example twenty-five peanuts) before they begin free eating. Dr. Jain does not require the super challenge because he found that most of his patients had a difficult time with the amount of allergen they had to eat for it. He found that it was very safe and much simpler for them to gradually incorporate the food into their diets at home.

Graduation gives patients and families "food allergy freedom" in the sense that the patient has bite-proof protection, which is a major milestone. This means that the patient can eat in restaurants and attend public events where their allergen is served. As long as the food is not a major ingredient of the dish that the patient consumes, the risk of reaction from small amounts or cross contamination is very low. Furthermore, if the patient consumes the OIT maintenance dose daily without a reaction, it signals the immune system that the food is not dangerous and the tolerance continues to improve. In approximately six months to one year, the threshold at which the patient can have a reaction increases to such an extent that the patient is considered to have "free eating status."

However, free-eating status does not mean persistent or sustained tolerance, since they have several years of daily maintenance dosing before they can reduce the frequency of exposure to twice a week.

OIT Maintenance Phase (Three+ Years)

During maintenance, patients continue to take their maintenance dose every day (at least initially) and, depending on their protocol, may be otherwise free to eat their allergens. At this point, some patients who had been dosing twice a day are able to switch to dosing once a day. Also, some doctors (including Dr. Jain) allow most patients to gradually reduce the observation and rest periods after dosing.

My daughter switched from taking her nuts twice a day to taking them once a day, which was a huge relief for us. We also dropped her rest period, allowing her to have a Snickers bar right before a gymnastics class (for extra energy). I also now occasionally give her peanut butter and jelly sandwiches for her lunch at school or camp.

Maintenance dosing can be challenging, however, as now patients are eating relatively large quantities of their allergen. Even people who like peanuts can get sick of eating them every single day. Maintenance is especially challenging for people who have done oral immunotherapy for multiple foods. My daughter, for example, did oral immunotherapy for peanuts, five tree nuts, and buckwheat. Her daily OIT maintenance dose consisted of the following:

- Five peanut M&Ms or roasted peanuts
- Three hazelnuts
- One-half pecan
- One-half walnut
- Four pistachios
- One, and a half cashew
- Four large buckwheat crackers (or five large capsules filled with buckwheat flour)

It was a slog to get her to eat these foods every single day. I completely exhausted my creativity in coming up with new recipes that use all these foods. Our biggest success was "multi-nut pancakes," but she started hating those too after less than a week. For the first year, we stuck to plain nuts, which is her preference because the quantity is smaller. She took her nuts while watching TV, which did help with the complaining. Even so, it was not easy for either of us.

Maintenance is easiest for people who treat only a few allergens. The challenge of maintenance for multiple foods is one of the main reasons that some allergists (like Dr. Jain) prefer to use other treatments, like SLIT, for minor allergens.

One Saturday morning, about four months after reaching maintenance, my daughter breezed through her nuts and danced out of her bedroom, ready to join her brother playing outside. I didn't say anything, let her go, then went into her room. A few minutes later, I called her in. "Layla," I said, "what's this?" pointing to a pile of nuts hidden behind her bookcase, and she immediately began crying.

Twenty grams of nuts every day is a lot for a small child. I don't know of a single kid who has gone through OIT and now eats that many nuts happily every single day. Milk is easier on my son, who gulps his 120 mL happily morning and night and sometimes asks for more.

After a few months—and after a long discussion with Dr. Jain—we decided to try moving my daughter to every other day dosing. This worked for a few weeks, and then she had a minor reaction to a dose. We switched back to every day dosing for another few months. After a few more months, we tried again to switch to every other day dosing, and this time were successful. There have been some twists and turns along the way as we figured out a doable maintenance dosing schedule but we are now at a stable point. We divide her nuts into two groups, and she doses peanut, cashew, and pistachio on the first day and hazelnut, walnut, pecan, and buckwheat on alternating days.

Switching to every-other-day dosing is a huge improvement in the quality of life for everyone I know who has made the switch, even though there is some additional risk involved if your child's body isn't quite ready.

It is worth staying in contact with your allergist and scheduling follow up consultations so that you might consider if/when you and your child may be ready to move toward every other day dosing.

Sustained Tolerance

Sustained tolerance is the dream we all want for our allergic kids. It means that your child can now freely eat their former allergens as much (or as little) as they like, and the allergy won't come back even if you stop maintenance dosing. My kids aren't there yet, but we hope that they will be in the next few years (perhaps even by the time this book is published).

Sustained tolerance seems to mimic what happens in the body when a food allergy is naturally outgrown. This is pretty close to the "cure" of which we have all dreamed. Sustained tolerance has been studied in clinical trials, with patients avoiding their allergen for several months after completing the updosing phase of OIT and then challenging it again after that period. Studies suggest that sustained tolerance is uncommon after only six months of maintenance and most frequently achieved after about three years of maintenance.

Skin tests and blood tests can provide good indicators of when sustained tolerance is reached. Throughout the updosing and maintenance phases of OIT, skin tests and blood tests still show positive results. But with time, the results become less strong and eventually, become negative. There is also another marker, called IgG4, which eventually increases, and that is a good possible indication of sustained tolerance.

When this happens, some allergists allow you to stop daily and/or every-other-day dosing. The food should still be eaten regularly, incorporated into the diet at least two to three times a week. This is the same recommendation as for foods that are naturally outgrown. Other OIT doctors prefer to err on the safe side and recommend daily maintenance dosing for life, or at least until further studies are done. It is true that sustained tolerance is still a relatively new research area, and it is not entirely clear that all patients will reach sustained tolerance. However, in Dr. Jain's experience, it is really just a matter of time for most patients.

The decision as to whether or not to stop daily maintenance dosing is one that will depend on the patient, the doctor, and the family. Personally, I did not want my kids to have to eat their allergens every day for life. That did not sound like the freedom that I wanted for them. It was only after I learned that some doctors do not require "daily maintenance for life" that I began to consider OIT as an option for my kids. It may mean additional risk for our family but I personally would prefer to manage a small amount of risk and have total and complete food allergy freedom without a requirement to eat certain foods every day for the foreseeable future. When my kids are old enough, the decision of whether/how they want to incorporate their allergens into their diet will be their decision, not mine. My hope is that by that time they will have had sustained tolerance for a number of years.

Chapter 6:

Special Considerations with OIT

Dairy OIT

Dairy allergies are becoming more common, and many parents find managing them to be quite difficult. Wheat and egg are the other two with this reputation. As a parent, I was comfortable managing allergies to peanuts, tree nuts, fish, and buckwheat. Discovering my son's milk allergy was the one that pushed me to desperation. Milk allergies are *hard*. Milk is everywhere in our society, far more common than even the ubiquitous peanut. Almost all social events in the United States involve pizza, cake, ice cream, pastries, or other foods with milk in them.

There are two types of milk proteins, casein and whey, and your child may be allergic to one or both of them. Whey proteins break down under heat, while casein stays stable. About 75 percent of kids with dairy allergy can tolerate baked milk. This means that they can have cakes, cupcakes, muffins, and other baked goods that have been baked for at least thirty minutes at 350 degrees F or higher.

If your child can tolerate baked milk, you can greatly increase the chances of them outgrowing the allergy by regularly giving him baked milk. Studies have shown that almost all children with a milk allergy who tolerate baked milk and eat it regularly outgrow the milk allergy within a few years. Thus, if you are willing to wait, you may not need treatment to rid your child of their milk allergy.

If you don't know if your child can tolerate baked milk, an allergist can perform skin prick and/or blood tests to look at responses to the different milk proteins. While these tests are important and helpful, they are also not always accurate, and a baked milk challenge is an important next step if the allergist believes your child is a good candidate. If the allergist thinks the blood test numbers and skin prick results are too high to warrant a test or you fail the baked milk challenge (as my son did), then you may wish to seek other types of treatment for the allergy.

OIT is the most common treatment for dairy allergy and can be done with baked milk or uncooked milk. Treating an anaphylactic milk allergy is considered to be especially hard, relative to other allergens. Most OIT is two steps forward, one step back, but milk OIT is two steps forward, two steps back almost as often. Many patients in milk OIT get stuck at some point, meaning that they cannot seem to updose beyond a certain amount without symptoms. As a result, the typical time to complete milk OIT is generally about double the time to complete immunotherapy for other foods. And reactions along the way are more common. While milk OIT can be hard, that isn't to say it isn't worth it. Unlike many foods, most children are happy to take their milk doses, and they can be taken in many different forms (whole milk, chocolate milk, yogurt, ice cream, etc.).

Baked Milk OIT

Baked milk OIT is what we did with Asim, first building tolerance for baked milk before tackling uncooked milk. The advantage is that it can be lower-risk than uncooked milk, and it opens up many possibilities for diet expansion along the way. However, most allergists agree that it is not required and that skipping baked milk and going straight to uncooked milk OIT makes for a faster total treatment.

My son, who failed the baked milk challenge at one-eighth of a cupcake, started baked milk immunotherapy with one-eighth of a cupcake. We gradually increased the dosage until he was eating the equivalent of two full cupcakes every morning. Once your child has been tolerating baked milk for a while, you can challenge baked cheese. We gave my son pizza for the first time on New Year's day 2016, and not only did he pass the challenge, but he loved the pizza. We now have pizza for dinner every Saturday night. It is amazing how much a little thing like pizza can improve your quality of life.

Once my son was regularly eating baked cheese, we got permission to give him uncooked butter and cream. Uncooked butter and cream only have miniscule amounts of protein in them (their labels read 0g protein, but that doesn't mean that there is actually none). While this tiny amount is enough for some people to have serious reactions, Dr. Jain told us that almost everyone who can have pizza can have butter and cream. Butter and cream also mean that most frosting is now ok. So we could bring my son to birthday parties, let him eat the pizza, and even the cake. The only exceptions are cake with cream-cheese frosting, which has only been offered once at all of the birthday parties and other celebrations I have been to in the past year.

If you start with baked milk OIT, once your child is tolerating pizza for a while, you can challenge uncooked milk. Your child may not be able to freely drink uncooked milk, but they may be able to tolerate a small amount. We challenged my son a few months after he started eating pizza, and he was able to tolerate 15 mL of uncooked milk. That became the starting point for uncooked milk OIT.

Uncooked Milk OIT

If you deicde to do uncooked milk OIT, by the time you get to about 20 mL, you can do an oral challenge for baked milk (this is assuming that your child could not tolerate baked milk prior to starting OIT). Most kids who can tolerate about 20 mL of uncooked milk can also tolerate baked milk. Remember that, if you choose to begin OIT with uncooked milk and are struggling, you can reconsider baked milk OIT.

Following baked milk OIT, we began uncooked milk OIT. Many patients do well with uncooked milk OIT, zooming through with no symptoms. That was not our experience. My son got all the way up to 120 mL of milk tolerated, the final dose under Dr. Jain's protocol, before he started reacting. His reactions were severe enough that we had to drop him down all the way to 30 mL. It then took us months to be able to increase the dose because just 35 mL would give him hives. After months of backtracking and then building back up, my son now drinks 120 mL again daily.

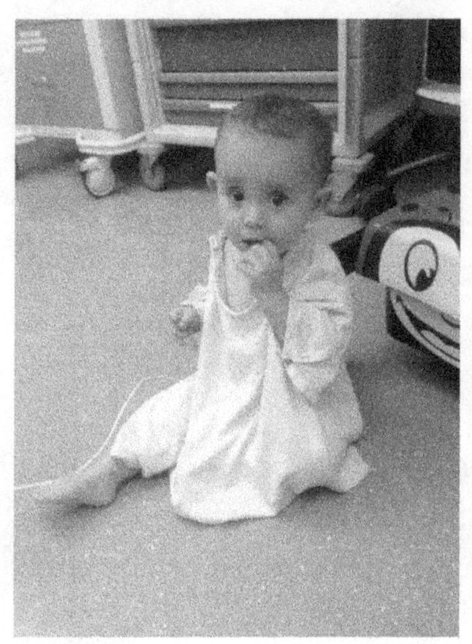

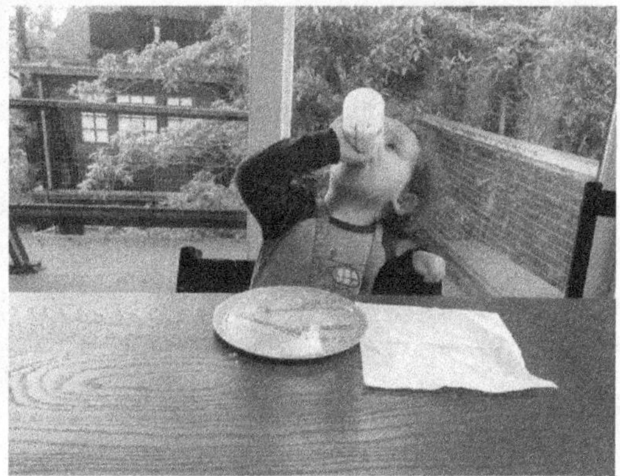

The author's son had his first trip to the ER (left) when he was only eleven months old. Here he is just over year later (right), now chugging real cow's milk.

Multiple Food OIT

More and more often, allergists are offering multiple food OIT, which means treating multiple foods all at the same time. It is frequently offered for similar "types" of foods (e.g., treating all tree nuts together), but treatment is increasingly available even for types of foods that are not so similar (e.g., milk and eggs, nuts and seeds). Dr. Jain has helped to pioneer the use of multiple food OIT (sometimes called mOIT).

My daughter did mOIT for peanuts and five tree nuts (hazelnuts, pecans, walnuts, cashews, and pistachios). With mOIT you start with a small dose of each allergen, which may or may not be mixed together.

My daughter's doses were mixed and all at the same starting dose. She started with 0.1mg of each of her six nuts (0.6mg total). When you do mOIT, you may not know which of the allergens caused a reaction, so you decrease all of the doses if that happens. I like to think of mOIT as being limited by your worst allergen and all of the others getting a free ride through treatment.

Amazingly, my daughter didn't have any severe reactions while doing mOIT. She did have a few minor reactions. For example, she got hives at 0.15 grams of each nut, which caused us to maintanin that dose for an extra week before returning to updose all of her nuts. We didn't know which nut had caused her reaction, and we didn't need to.

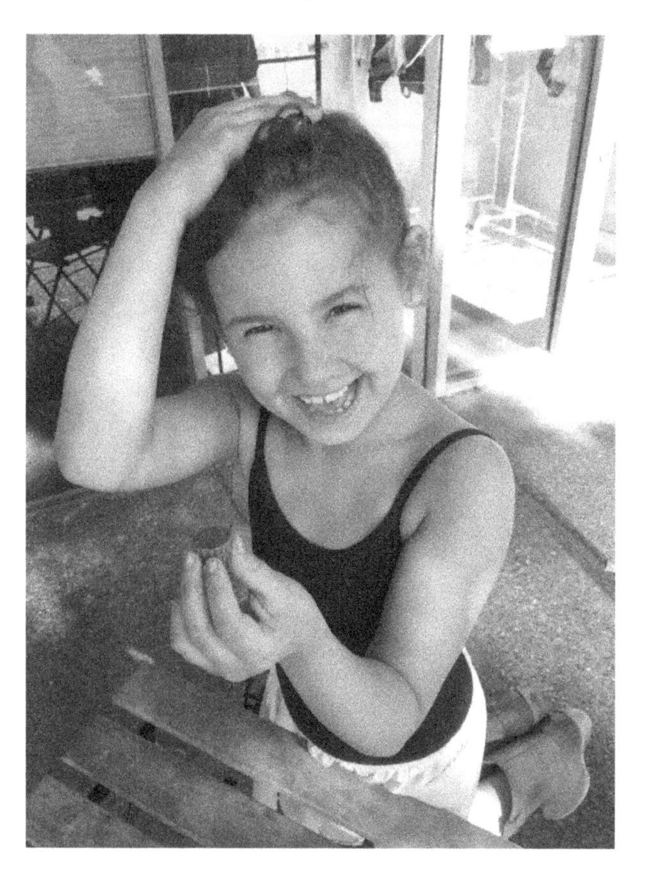

The author's daughter, age six, having her first ever Reece's Peanut Butter Cup

Peanut Pill

In late January 2020, the FDA approved Aimmune Therapeutic's Palforzia, the first and only food allergy treatment to receive this designation to date. This treatment, sometimes known as the "peanut pill," is a standardized pharmaceutical-grade dose of peanut protein in a capsule form.

Similar to standard OIT, initial dosing is done in an allergist's office under the observation of trained healthcare staff. The capsule is broken open and added to soft food to be taken by mouth. Once stabilized on a certain dose, the patient is sent home to continue that dose and procedure until the next appointment. All updosing appointments take place in an allergist's office under observation.

So what are the advantages and disadvantages of using a pharmaceutical product versus custom OIT treatment? The biggest advantage of Palforzia is that, in order to get FDA approval, it had to demonstrate a pharmaceutical grade of precision, have highly controlled (and expensive) manufacturing processes, and include a standardized protocol. This may provide medical doctors, parents, and patients with more comfort with and reassurance about the process of oral immunotherapy. This, in turn, may lead to expanded access as more allergists are willing to offer food allergy treatment. Another possible advantage is that as a FDA-approved drug, treatment may be covered by insurance.

The first disadvantage of Palforzia relative to custom OIT is that it is only available for peanut allergies. Second, the starting dose of Palforzia is considerably higher than the starting dose in custom OIT. If the patient reacts to the first dose, the doctor will either have to dilute the dose (which is not part of the FDA approved protocol) or discontinue treatment. This may pose some risk in the hands of doctors who have not had experience with custom OIT protocols and methods. A final disadvantage is cost. While treatment may be covered by most insurance plans, with a list price of $890 per month, the cost of Palforzia far exceeds the cost of peanuts in custom OIT. Overall, while Palforzia aids in creating a more standardized and pure product, there is less flexibility for patients who are unable to work within the strict parameters approved by the FDA.

OIT with Biologics

For patients with more severe or complicated allergies, combining biologic agents with oral immunotherapy may greatly improve efficacy and speed of treatment. The most commonly used biologic is Xolair (omalizumab). Xolair is an injectable antibody drug approved to treat moderate to severe allergic asthma by blocking the activity of IgE. When used in conjunction with OIT, it is given by injection every two to three weeks and costs about $2,000 per dose. Another biologic, Dupixent (dupilimab) is also being studied in clinical trials.

Studies have demonstrated that Xolair can speed up the OIT process, reduce side effects, and increase the amount of allergen a patient can tolerate. Based on data from seven clinical trials, the FDA designated Xolair as a breakthrough therapy and accelerated the approval process for treating food allergies. Dupixent is in phase 2 trials for food allergy treatment. Combining OIT with biologics is a promising area, although it is not widely available as a treatment option at this point. The FDA has approved these biologics for other indications: omalizumab for asthma and chronic hives; and dupilimab for asthma, nasal polyps, and eczema. However, they are not currently approved by the FDA for the treatment of food allergies. They are quite expensive and unaffordable for most patients if not covered by insurance.

CHAPTER 7:

Sublingual immunotherapy (SLIT)

The next food allergy treatment is sublingual immunotherapy (SLIT). SLIT is the regular administration of gradually increasing doses of allergens, delivered via drops under the patient's tongue, to achieve tolerance. It has been around for more than forty-five years, and its safety profile makes it an attractive option for many people. SLIT is widely used to treat environmental allergies using the same extracts as for allergy shots. While commercially made extracts are available for certain foods (the same extracts used in skin prick testing), though, SLIT is not a common treatment method for food allergies. Far fewer allergists offer SLIT than provide OIT, and many doctors have a negative impression of SLIT as being ineffective and/or slow.

The lack of SLIT availability stems in large part to its history of being used by ear, nose, and throat doctors at low doses where its efficacy has been questionable. In addition, the effects of SLIT are less robust than that of OIT, and so much larger sample sizes are needed in research studies to detect its effects. Performing carefully designed and monitored large clinical trials is very expensive and, so far, no pharmaceutical company has pursued such studies for FDA approval. As a result, there are fewer clinical trials and scientific papers that include SLIT in their scope. However, it is being used in select allergy private practices and is a great treatment option for many people.

How SLIT Works

In SLIT, the site of action is the mouth, rather than the gastrointestinal track as in OIT. You hold drops containing low concentrations of your allergen under your tongue, and the allergen is taken up by dendritic cells to the lymph nodes. There, it activates the regulatory arm of the immune system and dampens allergic activity. Under the tongue is a special area because it has a high concentration of dendritic cells and high permeability to large molecules such as proteins. This is important because dendritic cells "present" an allergen to the immune system and can either induce tolerance or an allergic state.

With SLIT, the regulatory arm of the immune system sees the allergen and works to calm the system and return it to baseline. The key is to find the therapeutic window or a dose that is large enough to activate the regulatory arm of the immune system—but not so large that it activates the stimulatory pathway. By gradually increasing the concentration of allergen in the drops, the immune system is learning to tolerate greater amounts of the allergen over time. It is important to recognize that the immune system only understands the language of concentration of the antigen or allergen. For this reason, even though the individual is receiving a very small amount of the allergen, which makes the process safe, the local concentration is high enough to lead to a much greater level of tolerization than what would be predicted from the amount of protein administered.

When to Use SLIT

SLIT has traditionally been seen as a bridge to OIT, useful when a patient is unable to tolerate the lowest starting dose. In these cases, a course of SLIT increases tolerance and usually allows OIT to follow. However, SLIT might make sense as a standalone treatment in certain situations.

Young Children

The first situation is in very young children. OIT is often not started until about two to six years of age. Doctors want patients to be able to reliably communicate what they're experiencing, and children younger than two generally do not have that capacity. As SLIT is much less likely to cause adverse effects, allergists may be comfortable starting treatment at a younger age. As an added bonus, since younger children have more malleable immune systems, they may be more likely to get all the way to free eating with SLIT alone, even for major allergens.

Minor Allergens

Minor allergens are foods that a patient is allergic to but maintain some tolerance. Perhaps their reactions are not severe (e.g., itching, hives, or stomachache), or they can tolerate a relatively large amount of the food before they start to react. In many of these instances, SLIT might lead to tolerance and allow free eating.

Delayed-Type Allergic Reactions

Some medical conditions such as atopic dermatitis (AD) and eosinophilic esophagitis (EOE) represent delayed reactions that are primarily cell mediated instead of antibody mediated. The regulatory arm of the immune system can suppress these reactions just as well as it can dampen IgE mediated reactions such as hives, swelling, or anaphylaxis. SLIT, therefore, has the potential of treating conditions such as AD and EOE. Dr. Jain has treated many patients with these conditions using SLIT. In general, the treatment protocol is prolonged and is not reliably successful. However, in patients where it is successful, the impact is quite dramatic in that patients can get relief without allergen avoidance and the use of chronic medications.

Safety/Protocol Concerns

SLIT protocols tend to be easier to manage and have greater compliance and fewer adverse effects than OIT. For those with safety or management concerns, SLIT might be a more attractive option, especially if the desired result is protection against cross-contamination or becoming "bite proof" rather than free eating or sustained tolerance. It might also be an attractive option for those with multiple allergies or fairly uncommon allergies. As mentioned previously, one of the biggest challenges with OIT is the long tail of maintenance. It can be difficult logistically and emotionally to eat a daily maintenance dose of a combination of different foods and/or foods that most people do not eat on a daily basis. The ability to mix multiple allergens into one bottle of drops and get protection through a couple squirts under the tongue may be very appealing. Yes, your child might not get all the way to free eating through SLIT, but you might avoid many emotional meltdowns and power struggles along the way. And there is some reason to believe that long-term SLIT maintenance might lead to increased tolerance over time.

Dr. Jain's SLIT Protocol

Most food SLIT protocols in the United States have grown out of Allergy Associates of La Crosse. At La Crosse, allergists have been treating patients with SLIT for both environmental and food allergies since 1970, and there is a strong track record of success. The La Crosse Method is individualized to the patient and their needs. However, their protocol includes dosing three times per day, and the average course of treatment is three to five years. They believe in dosing at lower levels more frequently and for a longer period of time. The main complaints with the La Crosse Method are that treatment is slow and that the goal is to build enough tolerance that accidental exposure wouldn't cause a significant life-threatening reaction, rather than getting to free eating.

Dr. Jain has developed a SLIT rush desensitization protocol that allows treatment to progress much more quickly. In his standard protocol, there are four treatment bottles of drops (labeled green, blue, gold, and red, these designations likely differ in other practices). Each bottle has five times the concentration of allergen protein as the previous bottle. Patients progress through sixteen levels of increasing doses (four levels for each of the four bottles) over the treatment phase. Once they reach the highest dose of four pumps of the red bottle, they will continue this maintenance dose at home for at least thirty days and then proceed to the next course of treatment. SLIT drops are temperature-sensitive, so they must be kept refrigerated at all times.

In addition to commercially available extracts of common allergens, Dr. Jain's staff prepares custom extracts to cover virtually any food allergy. These custom extracts are produced in a commercial kitchen but do not have the same level of precision and quality controls as a pharmaceutical-grade product. In his experience, though, the concentration of protein is low enough in SLIT that it does not really matter. Up to twenty different allergens can be desensitized at once in Dr. Jain's standard SLIT protocol.

The decision about whether to desensitize to multiple foods at once will be determined in discussions with your allergist prior to starting treatment. There is an obvious cost and time benefit if you can combine multiple allergens into one SLIT bottle. With that said, Dr. Jain does not mix severe and more minor allergens together as there is the risk of a reaction to the severe allergen increasing sensitization to the minor allergens. For example, if your child has severe peanut and tree nut allergies and more minor allergies to wheat and soy, you might combine the wheat and soy into one bottle and do SLIT for those separate from SLIT for the peanut and tree nuts.

The Black Bottle

Dr. Jain's standard SLIT protocol involves sixteen dosing levels with four bottles of drops. In certain situations, patients will be treated with four additional levels of dose increases. A black SLIT bottle has five times the concentration of allergen protein as does the red bottle. Instead of stopping at four pumps of the red bottle, patients would then updose from one to four pumps of the black bottle. Similar to the standard protocol, once at four pumps of the black bottle, patients maintain that dose for at least thirty days before moving on to the next phase of treatment.

You might be asking when and why a patient would want or need the black bottle instead of stopping at the red bottle. Theoretically, using the black bottle is always better in the sense that tolerating that higher level of allergen is related to greater desensitization. Rather than a daily dose of approximately 2mg of protein, those using the black bottle receive five times that amount every day. Patients who use the black bottle are more likely to pass an oral challenge or are able to start OIT at a higher dose. This might be very helpful for those with severe allergies, while it perhaps is unnecessary for those whose allergies are not as severe.

The primary downsides to using the black bottle are logistical and financial. On the logistical side, you can only desensitize four allergens per black bottle versus twenty in the red bottle. There is a limit to how much protein can be held in suspension, and the black bottle is five times more concentrated than the red bottle. On the financial side, there is the time, energy, and cost of additional updosing appointments.

Dosing Appointments

SLIT appointments are similar to those for OIT. They can be long days (depending on how many updoses you do), so prepare yourself and your child accordingly. All the tips and tricks I covered in chapter 5 work here.

When a patient arrives at the office, they are shown into a room where they will spend the next one to four hours, on average. You will be asked about any recent illnesses or changes in health, and your child's vital signs will be taken. If everything looks good, a nurse will administer the first dose, one pump of drops of the green bottle. Your child will hold the dose under their tongue for one to two minutes before swallowing. Most children tolerate the drops very well and say they taste sweet. Vital signs are monitored for twenty to thirty minutes after the dose, and if there is no reaction, they increase to two pumps. Again, the patient is monitored for twenty to thirty minutes before updosing to three pumps, and then to four pumps after another observation period. Dr. Jain typically stops after four updoses, even if there are no symptoms. If any reaction does occur, updosing is stopped and a patient will typically stay at the dose they had before the reaction occurred.

This is the protocol that will be used when you return to the office for updosing appointments. You will bring your current bottle of SLIT with you, kept cool with an ice pack. Once the patient reaches four pumps of a given bottle, they move to one pump of the next bottle (which has a higher concentration of protein). By doing this, a patient will move through the sixteen levels of SLIT doses in Dr. Jain's standard protocol. If using the black bottle, there will be twenty dosing levels.

In Dr. Jain's practice, the doctors and patients decide together how frequently to schedule updosing appointments based on the clinical needs of the patient and logistics (missing school/work, cost, etc.). Some choose to come in two to three times per week and move rapidly through treatment while others choose weekly or biweekly appointments. One of the benefits of SLIT is that the protocol is fairly flexible and most patients are able to progress through it quite rapidly if they want to.

At Home Dosing

Whatever highest dose your child reaches during an appointment will be their at-home dose until the next appointment. Doses should be taken at the same time of day. You cannot eat or drink anything for thirty minutes following a dose, and an observation period of one hour is highly suggested. During this observation period, the patient should avoid exercise, a hot bath/shower, or any activity that raises body temperature or increases heart rate. It is recommended that these activities be avoided for thirty minutes prior to taking the dose, as well.

Minor reactions do occur but are not as common as with OIT. Serious reactions are very rare. In general, SLIT is a more gentle treatment and is well tolerated. Of course, there is always a risk of a more severe reaction, so vigilance and proper monitoring of your child is important.

Communication with your allergist's office is key if there are reactions or if your child develops an illness or has a dental issue. For common colds without fever, you might be advised to reduce the dose by one pump and then add it back once the illness has passed. It is also typical to reduce the dose if your child has a loose/lost tooth or injury to the mouth or lips. Your doctor will work with you to determine how to handle these situations.

Maintenance Dosing

Once the patient reaches the highest dose of four pumps of the red or black bottle (which is about 2mg of allergen protein for the red and 10mg for the black), they will continue this dose at home for at least thirty days. What comes next is determined by the patient and their individual situation. Some may choose to undergo an oral challenge to the allergen as soon as possible. When more than one allergen has been included in the SLIT bottle, oral challenges are performed on different days so only one food is being tested at a time. Many patients, especially those with more minor allergens, are able to pass an oral challenge and introduce the food into their diet at that point.

Other patients may need to continue SLIT maintenance for a longer period of time before passing an oral challenge or progressing to OIT. Some may choose to stay on maintenance SLIT dosing for an indeterminate amount of time. This might be the case if the goal of treatment is to protect against severe reactions and the food is not one that is easy to eat on a daily basis. For example, say your child has a shellfish allergy and you want protection against cross-contamination and accidental exposure and you are fine with shellfish not being a regular part of their diet. Ongoing SLIT maintenance might be a low hassle way of keeping the desensitization gains made during treatment.

CHAPTER 8:

Epicutaneous Immunotherapy (EPIT)

Epicutaneous immunotherapy (EPIT), better known as patch therapy, works by increasing tolerance to a food allergen through the skin. It is far less widely used than OIT or SLIT, and few allergists in private practice offer this treatment. This may be due, in part, to EPIT having smaller effect sizes than OIT and SLIT. The goal of EPIT is protection from accidental exposures to a known food allergen. It is not designed to get someone to free eating status or sustained tolerance. The vast majority of food allergy patients are able to tolerate OIT or SLIT and would like the greater levels of desensitization that these treatments offer. However, for some, EPIT may be a necessary starting point for other treatments. And, for some, it may be a good standalone option that is lower risk (and also lower potential reward).

How Does EPIT Work?

When food is in contact with unbroken skin for a prolonged period of time, it activates the regulatory pathway of the immune system and dampens allergic activity. If the skin is injured, then contact with the allergen can activate the stimulatory arm of the immune system and lead to an allergic reaction. For this reason, placement of the patch is important and may be changed during treatment if the skin becomes damaged.

Similar to how SLIT works, in EPIT the allergen is taken up by specialized dendritic cells called Langerhans cells to the lymph nodes. There, it activates regulatory T cells and over time can induce desensitization. In contrast to the mouth, which has an extremely high concentration of antigen-presenting cells, the skin has fewer. Furthermore, skin is much less permeable to proteins than the lining of the mouth, and therefore, less allergen is accessible to the antigen-presenting cells. This helps explain why EPIT shows more modest effects in terms of how much protein can be tolerated after treatment, as compared to SLIT.

In general, someone who has undergone EPIT can usually tolerate about three to four times the amount of allergen protein after treatment as they could at the beginning. If the patch is worn for an extended period of time (more than a year), the effects appear to accumulate and increased tolerance is seen. Although this is positive, it is highly unlikely that anyone would see the same outcomes with EPIT as they would with SLIT or OIT. As such, in Dr. Jain's practice, EPIT is most often used as a bridge to one of these other treatments.

When to Use EPIT

Most people who use EPIT first attempt SLIT and cannot tolerate the starting dose. EPIT is also incredibly helpful as a first-line treatment for those with a credible history of anaphylaxis to an airborne allergen. In both of these cases, a course of patch treatment can increase tolerance enough that they can then progress to SLIT and possibly on to OIT from there. As I mentioned earlier, the skin has fewer antigen-presenting cells than the mouth does and is less permeable to allergens. This means that less protein will be absorbed through the skin, even if the same dose is used. However, custom EPIT also allows treatment with doses much lower than what is used in SLIT.

As an example, Dr. Jain had a patient who had an anaphylactic reaction to a very low dose of SLIT for her egg allergy. She was transitioned to EPIT, and once she was partially desensitized, she resumed SLIT and reached maintenance on egg SLIT. She is now undergoing OIT for her egg allergy. Another patient had an anaphylactic reaction from peanut being consumed by a person over ten feet from her. This patient was first started on EPIT then transitioned to SLIT, and over one year achieved a full maintenance dose of OIT. Now that patient has free-eating status for peanuts.

EPIT might be an attractive option for those who are looking for a relatively safe, well-tolerated, and easy treatment protocol. A company called DBV Technologies is counting on this. They are the makers of the Viaskin Patch, which you've probably heard about in the news.

The Viaskin Patch

DBV Technologies has developed a proprietary platform for delivering EPIT to patients ages four to eleven. Viaskin Peanut is in phase III clinical trials and has been designated as a Fast Track and a Breakthrough Therapy by the FDA. These designations are designed to accelerate the development and review of therapies used to treat serious conditions and fill an unmet need. In August 2019, DBV submitted a Biologics License Application to the FDA. Viaskin Peanut may become commercially available at some point. Viaskin Milk is in Phase II trials, and Viaskin Egg is in preclinical development.

Viaskin Peanut will use one standardized concentration of peanut protein, 250μg. It is expected that patients will purchase a monthly stock of patches and updose at home by wearing the patch for increasingly longer periods of time, rather than increasing the concentration of protein. Viaskin Peanut patches are to be changed every forty-eight hours.

Dr. Jain's Custom Patch Protocol

Dr. Jain has used custom EPIT for peanut, tree nuts, milk, egg, cinnamon, and chives and would be comfortable using it to treat virtually any food allergy. His protocol uses the same extracts he uses for SLIT. As a reminder, there are commercially available extracts for the most common allergens and then Dr. Jain's staff produces custom extracts in a commercial kitchen. This gives them much flexibility in terms of what allergens can be treated and with what doses.

Standard EPIT treatment in Dr. Jain's offices follows a similar protocol as described in the SLIT chapter. There are two treatment bottles, the latter with five times the concentration of proteins as the previous bottle. While the standard protocol works for most, it can be adjusted to meet individual patient's needs and sometimes requires more treatment bottles to accommodate a lower starting point. Each bottle can hold up to twenty allergens, allowing desensitization to multiple foods at once.

Patients begin with one pump of the first bottle and progress to four pumps before starting the next bottle in the series. There are eight total levels of escalating doses in the standard protocol. However, rather than the drops being held under the tongue as in SLIT, with EPIT they are applied to a patch which adheres to the skin. Patches are usually placed on the shoulder, the back, or the arms but can be placed virtually anywhere.

Dosing Appointments

When a patient starts EPIT, it is not a long appointment like OIT and SLIT. Only one updose is done in the office, as the allergen needs prolonged contact with skin to work. Similar to what has been described in earlier chapters, a dosing appointment will start with a staff member asking about recent illnesses or changes in health. They will also take vital signs to ensure that your child is in good health and ready to proceed.

The actual dosing consists of squirting one pump of the concentrate on the patch material and then placing this on the skin. The patient is monitored for twenty to thirty minutes to make sure there are no acute reactions to the dose. EPIT is generally well tolerated and has few serious side effects. The most common adverse reactions are redness, itching, and eczema. More generalized reactions have occurred but are extremely rare.

At Home Dosing

Patches are changed at home every forty-eight hours. Typically, patients increase their dose with each patch change until they have reached four pumps of whichever bottle they are on. If they develop eczema, the dose is lowered until it is controlled, and then they can resume updosing. Moving to the next treatment bottle is done in the office. There are no restrictions on activity or observation period with EPIT.

Maintenance Dosing

Once a patient has reached the highest dose, they will stay at that level for at least thirty days. The goal for most patients is to then transition to SLIT. Some might choose to do this immediately after the thirty-day period while others may stay on the maintenance dose for a longer time to increase the chances of making that transition successfully. In Dr. Jain's practice, few, if any, patients stay on EPIT for long-term maintenance.

Choosing Custom EPIT or Viaskin

Once Viaskin Peanut is FDA approved and commercially available, many allergists will likely begin offering this treatment. This is a huge advantage for many people who do not have local treatment options available to them. If your child has a peanut allergy and EPIT is of interest, this may be a great choice for you. Viaskin Peanut seems to be a safe and well-tolerated treatment and leads to a modest level of desensitization after fifty-two weeks of treatment.

Customized EPIT, available through select private practice allergists, would be a better option for those allergic to foods other than peanuts or those who would like to treat multiple allergens at the same time. DBV is pursuing EPIT for milk and eggs, but other allergens are not in the current pipeline. And many foods will likely never be. I think it is highly unlikely that Viaskin would offer an option to treat my daughter's buckwheat allergy, for example.

Additionally, because the Viaskin product is standardized, there is a possibility that some patients may react to the lowest dose commercially available. Dr. Jain's custom patches can start at a level that is 1,000 times lower than that offered by Viaskin. So while the Viaskin option will probably work well for most people, it may not be a good option for the most sensitive patients.

Chapter 9:

Chinese Herbs (FAHF-2)

The last evidence-based treatment is Food Allergy Herbal Formula-2 (FAHF-2). It was developed by Dr. Xiu-Min Li, who holds dual Professorships in the Department of Microbiology and Immunology and the Department of Otolaryngology at the New York Medical College (NYMC). Dr. Li maintains a robust research program, both in her lab at NYMC and in collaboration with colleagues at prestigious institutions in the United States, as well as medical schools in China. Her research focuses on the treatment of eczema, asthma, and food allergies with Chinese Herbs. As is always the case in clinical trials, what is being tested is a standardized protocol. Dr. Li also has a private clinical practice in New York where she treats patients with these conditions using customized protocols.

How FAHF-2 Works

Trained simultaneously in Chinese medicine and Western medicine in her native China, Dr. Li has a unique understanding of modern medicine, immunology, and Traditional Chinese Medicine (TCM) principles and practice. Using this dual perspective, she developed a nine-herb formula that targets food allergies called FAHF-2 based on a centuries-old formula for treating parasitic infections. This is based on the insight that the allergic mechanism in our bodies is designed to fight off parasites, as well as other pathogens. In the case of food allergies, our bodies are misdirecting this response toward certain proteins in harmless food.

FAHF-2 treats the whole immune system, tackling not only food allergens but also environmental allergens, asthma, and eczema. As such, it is a great option for people who have many issues that need treatment and would like a holistic approach. FAHF-2 works by stimulating the regulatory arm of the immune system and dampening allergic activity. The goal is to rebalance IgE and IgG in the immune system over time. The treatment initially seems to increase IgG4 production and inhibit activity of basophils and mast cells. The effects are like taking steroids but without the side effects. Over time, IgE levels begin to fall as memory cells stop producing allergy antibodies to specific foods. FAHF-2 is considered safe, is well-tolerated, and has had no serious adverse effects.

In mouse models, FAHF-2 completely blocks peanut-induced anaphylaxis. Subsequent research extended this to multiple food allergies, with FAHF-2 preventing anaphylaxis simultaneously to peanut, egg, and fish exposure. In these studies, FAHF-2 has been shown to be safe at many times the therapeutic dose.

These same effects have not yet been replicated in human studies. Dr. Li has speculated that this might be a dosing artifact, as humans would need to take thirty-six pills a day for two to three years to reach the same dosage as what the mice received in the studies. FAHF-2 was shown to be safe and showed immunological promise in the peripheral blood, but a substantial number of patients just could not keep up with the dosing requirements.

Dr. Li and colleagues continue to conduct research and refine the dosing, timing, and protocol of FAHF-2, as well as examining how to combine it with other treatments, to increase efficacy. FAHF-2 has now been refined twice, first with butanol to produce B-FAHF-2 and then with ethyl acetate, which is used to decaffeinate coffee and tea, to produce E-B-FAHF-2. These refinements separate the therapeutic compounds from the nontherapeutic ones and so reduce the volume of pills that patients must take, which was a burden in clinical trials for FAHF-2.

While a standalone clinical trial of the new version to support creation of a pharmaceutical drug must await the massive funding necessary, E-B-FAHF-2 is being studied at two sites as part of a triple therapy with omalizumab (Xolair) and multi-allergen OIT. It is hypothesized that the herbal therapy will reduce the adverse effects that are common with OIT and prolong desensitization. The goal of this treatment is to retrain the body so that it is no longer allergic (meaning it will not remember that it is allergic, whereas with OIT the immune system may never forget).

Dr. Li's Private Practice Protocol

In Dr. Li's private practice, she develops an individualized treatment plan for each client because most of them have comorbidities such as eczema, asthma, and allergic rhinitis and in some cases autoimmune disorders such as Crohn's Disease. Each plan typically includes specific herbs to take orally, as well as creams and herbal baths. The plan might also include acupressure and acupuncture. Versions of FAHF-2 and other FDA-registered Investigational New Drugs (IND) are used in her clinical practice, even without regulatory approval, because they are classified as dietary supplements rather than pharmaceuticals. Data collection is rigorous because, under a new FDA protocol, data from clinic-based "real world" studies are considered acceptable in lieu of double-blind placebo-controlled clinical studies. Parents of children who have done Chinese Herbs in private practice report fewer allergic reactions, less eczema, improved asthma, better digestion, and fewer illnesses overall.

Chinese Herbs were our first foray into food allergy treatment. I read about FAHF-2 before we started seeing Dr. Jain, and it appealed to me given the young ages of my children and the potential for broad-based treatment effects. We traveled to New York to see Dr. Li, and she started both of my children on regimens of pills, creams, and baths. After returning home, we had monthly follow-up phone calls over about a two year period. They both did well on the treatments, so no additional in-person appointments were needed.

Chinese Herbs protocols can be very challenging. At the height of my daughter's treatment, her protocol included cream all over her body twice a day: swallowing fifty pills per day (twenty-five in the morning and twenty-five in the evening) and a daily herbal bath with a twenty minute soak. Pill swallowing is not a talent; it is a skill that can be learned. We started with Nerds and progressed to Tic Tacs, Skittles, and then onto pills. At six years old, my daughter learned to swallow eight massive pills in a single gulp! Thankfully, though, by the time she was finishing her treatment, the total number of pills had decreased to about twenty per day.

As my kids grew older, we had more compliance issues with their FAHF-2 treatment plans. By that time, we were also doing SLIT and OIT, and their allergies and asthma were more under control. While I cannot definitively say what Chinese Herbs did versus the other treatments, I definitely believe there was an effect and that it contributed to our outcomes.

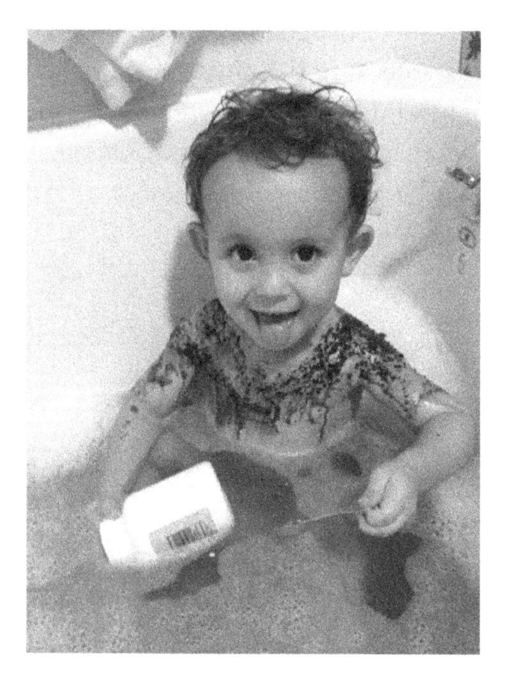

The author's son taking his daily FAHF-2 "herbal bath"

Accessing FAHF-2 Treatment

Until fairly recently, FAHF-2 was only available directly from Dr. Li and her team. Many families, like myself, made the trip to New York in order to become patients and access the treatment. Chinese Herbs are now available on the West Coast through Dr. Jain's practice. Dr. Yan Yan, in one of his Bay Area offices, was trained by Dr. Li and also received TCM training in China. She works closely with Dr. Li to develop and implement treatment plans without patients needing to travel to New York.

A cautionary note about Dr. Li's treatment versus Chinese herbal remedies you might find online or locally from an herbalist: Dr. Li's treatment, while using TCM herbs, has followed a scientifically rigorous western-style approach to testing. The herbs have a high level of quality control, which is not always followed by people selling herbs online or in a corner shop. A major cause of hospital admittances for liver damage is unregulated Chinese herbs, so quality control is extremely important. Dr. Li's team adheres to European standards (which are higher than American standards) to ensure the purity and quality of all ingredients used in their herbal formulas. You can read more about Dr. Li's work in the books *Food Allergies: Traditional Chinese Medicine, Western Science, and the Search for a Cure* and *Traditional Chinese Medicine, Western Science, and the Fight Against Allergic Disease.*

Chapter 10:

Combination Treatments

Some food allergies can be effectively treated with a single treatment. A good example of this is a severe peanut allergy that can be treated with OIT. Another example would be a handful of less severe food allergies that could be treated effectively with SLIT. However, for many, their allergies and treatment needs are not as straightforward. As a result, more and more doctors are increasing the number of treatment options that they offer in their portfolio.

Combining treatments can be challenging as the protocols, timelines, and cost become more complex. But combining treatments sometimes makes a lot of sense for more complicated cases. Both of my kids fell into the category of "complicated cases," and both went through combination treatments including OIT, SLIT, and FAHF-2. Described below are some of the more common experiences of combination treatments.

SLIT and OIT

SLIT and OIT is one of the most common combinations of treatments. SLIT is widely used as a means to introduce allergens to the most severe allergy patients, those who can't even tolerate the very first tiny dose of OIT. Many OIT allergists offer this as an option for their patients, but only if they discover that the first OIT dose was not well tolerated (which is rare).

Less common is the use of SLIT for minor allergens and OIT for major allergens. This combination was pioneered by Dr. Jain and is not yet commonly used by other allergists. The goal of Dr. Jain's protocol is to reduce the number of foods that require OIT. OIT for multiple foods can be extremely burdensome. In contrast, SLIT for many foods is relatively simple. My son is now in SLIT maintenance for forty-one foods, and those maintenance doses are far easier to manage than even just a single OIT food maintenance dose.

EPIT with SLIT or OIT

EPIT, or the Patch, increases tolerance for allergens less than other treatment methods and is unlikely to take someone to the point where they can free eat. For this reason, many patients prefer to combine it with additional desensitization methods. It is commonly used as a bridge to either SLIT or OIT for patients who cannot tolerate the lowest dose of one of those treatments or are having trouble moving forward. Patients who reach maintenance on EPIT may wish to switch to eating real food, rather than retain the patch for years of maintenance. After a challenge to determine how much they can tolerate post-EPIT, the patient can then increase the amount they eat until they are able to free eat their allergens. If they are not yet able to switch to real food after EPIT, continued Patch therapy or SLIT might be indicated.

EPIT and/or SLIT can also be used as a complementary treatment for OIT patients who have reached a resistance point and are having trouble moving forward. Dr. Jain finds that most patients have on average two to three resistance points while building on their OIT doses. Most of these patients simply need to slow down on their build-up protocol to overcome these resistance points. However, infrequently patients get stuck at a dose and simply do not make any progress for weeks or even months. In these instances, Dr. Jain and his colleagues have used EPIT, as well as SLIT, while maintaining a tolerated dose of OIT to break-through these barriers.

FAHF-2 with SLIT or OIT

FAHF-2 as a stand-alone treatment may not take patients to free eating for all of their allergens, in which case additional treatment may be desired. Both SLIT and OIT are good options depending on the severity of the allergies and treatment goals. While little has been published on these treatments in combination, both Dr. Li and Dr. Jain have seen excellent results in their patients.

FAHF-2 and SLIT is a wonderful combination that can take patients further than either treatment alone and yet still minimizes the risk of anaphylaxis. It is also a great combination for patients seeking to treat a large number of allergens, as SLIT can treat up to twenty allergens in a single vial, and there is no additional protocol challenge with having multiple vials (my son uses four SLIT vials). FAHF-2 treats *all* allergens with a single protocol. So SLIT plus FAHF-2 is a great combination for patients with a large number of allergens who may not get to free eating with SLIT alone.

FAHF-2 plus SLIT is still unlikely to take a patient with very severe allergies all the way to free eating, but it can happen. My daughter had a severe allergy to fish, with specific IgE>100, and a known history of reaction. Miraculously, SLIT plus FAHF-2 took her all the way to free eating. This is rare but possible.

There are several reasons to combine FAHF-2 with OIT. FAHF-2 can help OIT go more smoothly, reduce side effects, and bolster immunity overall. It can help patients if they are having a tough time getting past a resistance point. There is also some evidence that FAHF-2 may help reduce the duration of OIT maintenance dosing. Since for many people maintenance dosing is the most challenging part of OIT, anything that reduces the need for this can be worthwhile.

The main challenge of combining FAHF-2 with other treatments is the FAHF-2 protocol. SLIT drops are incredibly easy compared to the protocol challenges of FAHF-2. OIT falls into the middle in terms of protocol ease, meaning FAHF-2 plus SLIT will likely be easier than FAHF-2 plus OIT. Cost can also be a challenge, as FAHF-2 is generally considered the most expensive treatment. While both SLIT and OIT have a similar cost related to the active treatment phase, SLIT maintenance is considerably more expensive than OIT maintenance.

SLIT, OIT, and FAHF-2

Few patients are willing to manage the protocol requirements of combining SLIT, OIT, and FAHF-2. However, if one is able and willing to tackle this challenge, the combination of treatments can be very effective for the most complicated cases. Both of my kids fell into this category. Asim, with his forty-one food allergies, environmental allergies, and asthma, needed all of the treatment help he could get. My daughter had fewer food allergies, but we could not even imagine doing fish OIT for several different types of fish given the challenges of getting her to take maintenance doses for the other seven allergens she had.

With two kids in combination treatments, I developed an elaborate checklist for each medication that the kids had to take each day. Getting through this protocol for both kids every day was incredibly hard. For about a year, it was our top priority as a family, and we made numerous sacrifices to make it work.

Combination treatment became somewhat easier for Layla when she reached maintenance for OIT. She started taking her doses only once a day and later every *other* day. When we had protocol fatigue, Dr. Li told us that we could drop the baths and the creams and just keep the pills. About two years into treatment, Dr. Li also came out with her new FAHF-2 treatment protocol that had more concentrated pills, meaning Layla took fewer of them. Her total number of pills was then reduced from twenty-nine in the morning and twenty-nine at night to seventeen in the morning and ten at night.

About a year and a half into treatment, and at the challenging age of almost three, Asim stubbornly refused to take his herbs any more. Up until then, he had been relatively content to take them. We tried every method we could think of to get him to take them, but after a few weeks of struggling, we gave up. He still does his baths and creams but is no longer taking his pills.

Daily Medication Checklist for Asim and Layla	Sun	Mon	Tues	Wed	Thurs	Fri	Sat
MORNING							
Layla							
Cream III, light layer (blue)							
Zyrtec							
Breakfast							
OIT doses: buckwheat, peanuts, 5 tree nuts							
FAHF-2 pills (29 pills and capsules)							
Inhaler							
Brush teeth							
SLIT Drops (environmental and fish)							
Asim							
Cream IIIvb, light layer (green)							
Get dressed, use potty							
Breakfast							
5ml Zyrtec, mixed with FAHF-2							
Milk dose							
Brush teeth							
SLIT Drops 1 (environmental)							
SLIT Drops 2 (legumes, with dropper)							
SLIT Drops 4 (Commercial)							
SLIT Drops 4 (Asim custom)							
BEFORE NAP							
Asim							
Cream IIIvb							
EVENING							
Layla							
Bath with herbs							
Cream IIIvb, thick layer							
OIT doses: buckwheat, peanuts, 5 tree nuts							
Zyrtec							
Singulair							
FAHF-2 (29 pills and capsules)							
Brush teeth							
Inhaler							
Asim							
Bath with herbs							
Cream IIIvb, thick layer							
5ml Zyrtec, mixed with FAHF-2							
Milk dose							
Singulair							
Brush teeth							

Part III
Next Steps

Chapter 11:

Post-Treatment Life

You've read about each of the four treatments featured in this book and considered how they can be used alone and in combination. You've probably thought about your own child or loved one with allergies and what those protocols and investments would entail for all of you. And you've likely imagined what life might be like following treatment. After all, the primary reason people decide to pursue food allergy treatment is to improve safety and functioning in daily life. So what does life after treatment look like?

As you've read in my story and will see below in those of other families we've highlighted, most people who complete treatment find a new level of eating freedom that they did not enjoy previously. Social events like classroom celebrations, birthday parties, and potlucks are no longer dreaded and/or avoided. Kids are able to eat wherever they want during school lunches and can confidently go to a friend's house to play and hang out without bringing their own food. Families can eat out at restaurants and travel with an ease and spontaneity that was unthinkable before. Kids can enjoy Halloween and other holiday traditions openly and freely. Parents are less vigilant and anxious and stress levels decrease.

Life on the other side of treatment is wonderful. But it is not all fun and games. For many who complete treatment, there are new and unforeseen realities to accommodate and manage. For example, your child may need to take their daily nut dose at a "nut free" overnight camp. Or the challenge of having one child who has completed treatment and been told to continue eating the allergen every day, while a sibling is allergic and avoiding that same food. Many patients continue to have "mystery reactions" in maintenance. Part of the problem is that immunotherapy treats specific allergens but does not change a higher susceptibility to allergies and the possibility of an old allergy reemerging or a new one developing. For this reason, it is critical that emergency action plans continue to be updated and epinephrine carried at all times.

The stories included here, written in the first person narrative by either the patient or their parent, highlight the complexities of treatment and showcase how life after treatment can look. It takes bravery and grit to manage food allergies, and their treatment, and we are grateful to those who shared their journeys and experiences with us.

First patient to undergo multiple tree nut OIT

Two minutes. It is such a small amount of time. So small, in fact, that if I were told to wait two minutes, I might content myself to watch traffic or take that time to appreciate the weather. Often at work I find that many people use "two minutes" rather figuratively, often meant to indicate not that something will be done literally in one-hundred and twenty seconds but instead meant to communicate that not much time is needed. This all goes to show just how finite and small two minutes of time really is in my life, and I suspect it is equally small in the lives of others as well. Yet, in at least one instance of my life, two minutes was not used as a figure of speech; it was literally the amount of time I had between myself and a premature end.

I was not born with a food allergy. Instead, it is something that developed sometime in my prepubescent years, meaning that my first experience with these allergies was an unexpected one. On a September afternoon, my family and I made a stop by our local fast food restaurant, and I had tried a tiny sample of the candied walnut that my mom had bought. The next hour was normal, but on our drive home, I remember a heavy feeling in my chest, as well as pressure building in my throat. I wouldn't know it until later, but I was suffering from an anaphylactic reaction due to the candied walnut. My body is hyper allergic to tree nuts and in this case overreacted to the candied walnut and was in the process of closing my windpipe.

My parents, being the wonderful individuals they are, immediately rushed me to the hospital, where I remember seeing over a dozen medical staff pumping my body full of chemicals and antidotes. Eventually, the reaction began to subside, and my vitals stabilized, and that was when one of the doctors mentioned to my parents, verbatim, "Another two minutes, and we could not have done anything for him." Two minutes.

Now, as a young kid, I had to keep that knowledge at the forefront of my mind. Every family gathering, every time we went out to eat, even before having a candy bar, there were now some preliminary questions that were asked: Does this have tree nuts? Is there any risk of cross contamination? Do I have my medicine, and is there a hospital nearby in case I need treatment?

Maybe these questions sound paranoid, but under the threat of another anaphylactic reaction, they were very important and real. And, even despite the questions I'd ask, there was no guarantee that I would never be exposed again; the next two years of my life were filled with adjustments as my family and I adapted to our new normal. Sadly, that incident in September was not the last of my many hospital visits; the next few years, I went to the emergency room more times than I can recall. But what I do recall is being in the hospital after my third anaphylactic reaction and thinking that there had to be some other way of living. There had to be a solution to this. I just wanted to be able to live without having to worry about an accidental exposure resulting in a hospital visit.

Then I met Dr. Jain at Columbia Asthma and Allergy Center. It is important to note that I had multiple allergies as a kid, and I was visiting him for treatment regarding seasonal allergens at the time. However, upon learning of my situation, Dr. Jain proposed another treatment plan regarding my tolerance to tree nuts. It would be highly experimental, and the results weren't guaranteed, but it was possible that through the desensitization I could live a more normal life. I almost immediately agreed.

The treatment plan was based on exposure therapy. I would be given a small dose of jelly, which contained milligram quantities of seven common tree nuts, to be consumed twice a day. Over the course of several weeks, this dose would increase, giving me heightened immunity and decreasing the likelihood that I would need to visit the hospital if exposed to the allergens in the future. As with every experiment, there were some initial difficulties, but I never once felt unsafe or that I was in an uncontrolled environment. The desensitization was very intentional and methodic, which was something I did not learn to appreciate until years later.

As Dr. Jain and I went through the desensitization process, I eventually went from consuming jelly containing grams of the nuts to whole pieces of the allergens. This was a turning point for me; now, I held in my hand and could consume a concoction of nuts that would have only a year or two earlier killed me. And now I was able to consume them, albeit in a controlled and specific manner.

The treatment continued for years afterward, but at that moment something had really changed in my mentality and the way I thought about eating foods I hadn't personally prepared. I now felt a bit more trusting when I went out to eat and could enjoy the baked goods made by friends without having to worry as much about being exposed to tree nuts. That isn't to say the allergy went away completely; I still carry medicine to this day. But as someone with food allergies, I went from constantly worrying about exposure, to merely avoiding the tree nuts themselves. As you might imagine, this was liberating; I felt like I had a second chance at a more normal life.

The benefits from Dr. Jain's treatment still impact me today. I have had the privilege of serving in the US military and have traveled across many countries from Asia to the Middle East. And while abroad, I was able to partake in the local cuisines and treats, something I previously thought impossible. That isn't to say the allergy has disappeared entirely; in Vietnam I was almost forced to go to the hospital, in Thailand an accidental exposure caused much concern, and even in Seattle I had to take a few doses of Benadryl to stop an anaphylactic reaction. But the fact that the reactions could be handled and did not result in hospitalization or worse is a testament to the effectiveness of the treatment. Now, exposure is an inconvenience rather than a trip to the ER, and I can enjoy a variety of foods previously inaccessible.

And so, I want to dedicate these last few words to thanking Dr. Jain and those who made the treatment possible. You have provided me with a new quality of life that I previously didn't think was possible. If anyone else out there is suffering from severe food allergies, please understand that I know how much of a stressor it can be and how much it can weigh on your mind; but take it from me. There is hope, and there is a treatment.

SLIT for multiple food allergies

My son developed his first food allergy to dairy, through breastmilk, at three months of age. He then went on to develop allergies to egg at seven months along with cashew, pistachio, and pink peppercorn at seventeen months.

The first cashew reaction was incredibly scary. We were visiting friends, and he ate a cracker that was simply on a plate with cashew nut butter. His face started to break out in hives. I paged the on-call pediatrician as we administered Benadryl (at that time guidance didn't clearly recommend starting with epinephrine). She said we could simply wait and observe or, if we wanted to be more cautious, go wait in the ER parking lot. By the time we got there, my son was lethargic. His face and lips were swollen, and we watched the reaction progress down his body over the next few hours in the ER. Despite a steroid injection, his abdomen swelled up, and over the next few days, his skin peeled off as if he'd had a chemical burn. During our next visit to the allergist, we were advised to get rid of all nut and nut-containing products in our home and to practice strict avoidance.

Using my background in healthcare, I dove into the literature to educate myself. I was "that" parent. You might recognize my hypervigilance. I scoped out play structures for food left behind by other kids. I moved him away from kids who were eating. We took our own food and treats to birthday parties I deemed "safe enough" to attend after talking with the host. I offered to provide snacks for everyone when we had playdates and asked other parents not to bring any. I thought about food constantly. I called countless food manufacturers to ask about shared equipment. We grew to love our trusted allergen-friendly brands. I subscribed to the FDA's food recall notification service to monitor recalls among products we used. I worked with Dr. Jain to determine how to create a safe environment for my son at school and negotiated a food-free classroom. All kids washed or wiped their hands on their way into class to avoid surface contamination. And we focused on inclusion in all activities.

Despite my best efforts, we still had close calls. One day a friend who was very tuned into our needs was cooking for us. She went to scoop mustard out of a jar, and I saw white stuff on the spoon. What was it? It was mayonnaise that her husband had gotten into the mustard while making a sandwich.

Over the next few years, we saw several allergists, including some in major academic centers. We had one egg challenge in which they declared his egg allergy to be gone, only to have him experience a full-blown anaphylactic reaction two months later that required epinephrine, a 911 call, and a stint in the ER. Our retiring allergist suggested we see Dr. Jain. The best endorsement she could have given was mentioning she would take her own children to him.

I appreciated Dr. Jain's knowledge and patience in explaining things, his calm presence, and the lack of pressure to choose any one path. Despite that, it took me nearly a year to decide on a plan that felt comfortable in terms of both possible benefits and potential risks: SLIT for dairy and eggs, followed by SLIT for cashew and pistachio. We hoped to get to a point of being able to freely eat dairy and egg but, with cashew IgE scores over 100, only expected to reach a place at which cross-contamination was no longer a concern.

We chose an unusual path through SLIT, using higher doses than normal. We also continued SLIT maintenance for a long time before successfully challenging each item. My son now eats egg and dairy regularly. We were all pleasantly surprised when he passed both the cashew and pistachio challenges, eating one gram of cashews (about one and a half cashews) and five grams of pistachios (about eight pistachios). We decided simply to continue SLIT to build tolerance instead of progressing to OIT.

It took time to get used to our newfound freedom: buying foods without reading labels, ordering off the menu in restaurants without asking for the manager first, just walking into a restaurant without researching it first and calling ahead, going to friends' homes and eating whatever they offer without a bunch of discussion. Although we will always carry epinephrine because there are no guarantees, food allergies have become a distant memory for us. It has provided a tremendous sense of relief. And I no longer identify with the role of "food allergy mom!"

OIT for eggs and tree nuts and SLIT for environmental allergies

Our oldest son N was diagnosed with life-threatening food allergies to eggs and several tree nuts as a young infant. He also suffered from viral-induced asthma and chronic eczema. While tree nuts were somewhat easier to avoid, eggs were not, and we had basically resigned ourselves to living life in a protective bubble, declining any and all social events that involved food. We actually had no idea just how severe his egg allergy was until he went into anaphylaxis multiple times as a toddler. He was also contact sensitive to any egg-containing product, such as mayonnaise. After several random reactions that we couldn't pinpoint, we tested him for multiple foods when he was about ten months old. Interestingly enough, eggs did not even show up as an allergen. When we later decided to introduce egg because we thought it would be safe, he had a delayed reaction that awakened him from his nap involving full-body hives, eyes swelling shut, and vomiting. He was promptly transported to urgent care and given epinephrine. I will never forget the trauma of that first reaction.

Avoiding eggs was just a new way of life for us, and I became an excellent chef with incredibly creative substitutions. However, it became clear that it wasn't going to be safe for him to lead a normal independent life without constant supervision and worry. I was convinced homeschooling was the only way to keep him safe. I felt absolutely despondent, and I was weary and tired of explaining to well-intentioned parents that "yes, just a little could actually take his life." I was very fortunate that N was not a picky eater and ate an extremely healthy and varied diet and never developed a strong penchant for baked pastries, cookies, or cakes.

Luckily, I was well connected with our local parents' club, and a fellow mother with a daughter allergic to eggs informed us that her child was starting oral immunotherapy with one of the few Bay Area providers offering it in private practice (Dr. Jain) and was actually starting to tolerate egg in substantial quantities! While we had heard vaguely about OIT and the general idea of desensitization, we knew at that point it was only available in clinical trials for peanut. Our allergist at the time informed us to get in touch with Stanford to see if there might be something in the works for my child to participate in for the future. We were told by two separate allergists that our son's allergy was through the roof and he would likely never outgrow it (his IgE numbers were in the 300 range with equally glaringly positive skin-prick test results) and he would have to constantly be vigilant. We continued this way of life armed with our epinephrine and action plan until a conversation with an amazing mother in our local parent's group first gave us a glimmer of hope.

I am incredibly grateful for meeting this mother, who shared her child's struggles and success. I immediately called up the clinic after our conversation, and I was connected with a most delightful nurse. I spent about an hour speaking with her and trying to understand the process. She was calm, understanding, and exceptionally knowledgeable. I felt a huge weight lift off of my shoulders after our conversation and scheduled our consultation immediately.

At our first appointment, we met with Dr. Jain, who had a calm, confident presence and alleviated many of our concerns. He did convey to us that he had never observed numbers as high as our son's, but he was willing to start the desensitization process immediately. A few short weeks later, we began the process. Our son reacted to his very first dose of egg with eczema flares and hives on his arms. This was a 1:100 dilution of egg. We felt a lot of our initial hope slip away at that point, thinking he would never make progress. However Dr. Jain and his team came up with a plan to start at a much lower dose (1:1000) and customize his protocol to move slowly the following week. We proceeded with the cyclical process of weekly updosing, reactions, progress, illness, downdosing, followed by multiple setbacks over the next six months, and couldn't believe we actually made progress when we did. While it was a frustrating process for us, Dr. Jain remained unwavering and confident that N would eventually be able to eat eggs freely. Dr. Jain was always available to us via text/phone in the middle of the night to support us through reactions, and his dedication to his patients is admirable and rare.

Finally, in February of 2016, we were very excited when our son reached egg maintenance by tolerating a whole egg! However, the year following maintenance was still challenging because our son would still continue to react sometimes to his doses. He was losing teeth at that point which made him extra sensitive, so we had to modify our daily dosing to include even more egg when he was doing well, so he became further desensitized. After completing egg OIT at age four, we treated environmental allergies with SLIT, followed by multiple tree-nut OIT. He sailed through tree nut OIT and desensitized to five tree nuts over an insanely short period of three months without a single reaction during the updosing process. We believe that focusing first on his most severe allergen, followed by calming his immune system with environmental desensitization, facilitated the tree-nut OIT process.

Four years later, our son now continues to eat doses of an entire egg, plus eighteen grams of various tree nuts, on a daily basis. He is able to eat unlimited egg products, unlimited nut products, and his blood IgE numbers have fallen tenfold and have remained stable. His reactions have become fewer and far-between, and he has now taken on the responsibility of daily dosing on his own. We now don't have to read ingredient labels feverishly nor do we stress about traveling or having to find safe foods. We no longer worry that he is safe at school. His asthma flares and eczema are now completely controlled due to several years of allergy shots. Our family has been given this incredible gift of freedom, and we are so very grateful for finding Dr. Jain and the amazing staff at Columbia Asthma and Allergy clinic, who have been instrumental in improving the quality of life for our family! While the process can be lengthy, with patience and dedication, we believe others can find comfort in knowing their lives can also be transformed like ours!

Traveling out-of-state for SLIT and OIT treatment for multiple food allergies

My son J is seven years old. When he was one year old, he had his first allergic reaction. We learned he was allergic to peanuts, tree nuts, eggs and sunflower seeds. He outgrew the egg allergy, and we were able to start with baked eggs and then progress to regular eggs when he was three years old. We successfully avoided peanuts and tree nuts (hazelnuts, cashew, almonds, pistachio, walnut, pecan, macadamia, brazil nut) and sunflower seeds. In December of 2018, he had an anaphylactic reaction after eating turkey fried in peanut oil. He got an EpiPen immediately, and we were across the street from an emergency room. In less than ten minutes after ingestion he had an IV, steroids, Benadryl, Pepcid, and continuous albuterol nebulizers. But he continued to struggle to breathe. We ended up in a pediatric ICU overnight and multiple times they were preparing to intubate him but he avoided this. J had a history of a month long ICU stay when he was three years old due to a reactive airway that required nine days of intubation.

We began working with our allergist to try to find a way to make him less reactive. We did a bronchoscopy and EGD to make sure there wasn't an underlying issue. There wasn't, but he had bronchial spasms during it even though he was under general anesthesia. We tried Xolair, and after three shots, he had a reaction. I was meanwhile researching other options but being told he was "too reactive" or they could only do one allergen at a time.

I finally found Dr Jain, who did a phone consultation to review his records. Something he said that really struck me, and that I absolutely believe, was "Your son is too reactive to *not* pursue desensitization." He thought we should do SLIT and then OIT and that based on his history it might take a long time, maybe even years. But even some desensitization was going to be better than where we were now.

We live in Arizona, so starting treatment also meant travelling. We traveled to San Francisco in October during our fall break. We scheduled three office visits in different offices to be able to have three days of updosing. To our surprise, J finished SLIT, and we were able to start OIT during that week. Over the next few months, my son and I traveled every other week on Monday nights, spent Tuesdays in the Sunnyvale clinic doing updoses, and then flew out late that night. It was exhausting, but the clinic and staff really worked with us to make it possible. To our complete shock, in January we reached a "maintenance" dose of 2g of each nut or 20g of ground nuts (it fills a 2oz condiment container). As we were celebrating, J ran to give the doctor a hug and said, "Thank you for my freedom!"

So how has life changed? Freedom -- that word really sums it up completely. Before we started treatment, everything J ate was from a peanut/ tree nut free facility. I spent so much time researching, ordering, and trying to have a safe option ready for the "Oh, I forgot to mention ahead of time today in class/church/practice/party that we are having ______." He still carries an EpiPen, and he still could react if he accidentally ate a cookie or brownie with nuts in it. We are still careful. But he is now safe from cross-contamination and it makes all the difference in the world.

At the grocery store, I choose Valentine's Day treats based on what looks good, not what facility they were made in. I can complete a grocery store trip without a single search of manufacturers' websites/allergy information. J sits at the regular table at lunch and orders hot lunch when he wants it. He has now eaten at bakeries and ice cream shops. We spent a weekend at a Great Wolf Lodge, and I did not pack a single safe food/ treat (just his doses!). We have gone camping and been able to buy food locally because I didn't have to worry about brands/where they were processed. For family birthdays, I can order a cake at the local grocery store and not worry about it. We have flown on planes without having to pre-board and scrub down the seats ahead of time, wondering if this will be the time he reacts. He eats at so many restaurants that were previously off-limits because they used nuts in their kitchens. He has a newfound love for Dunkin Donuts! I had an entire pantry full of peanut/tree nut free facilities safe candies and treats and baking mixes and granola and crackers that I was able to give away. Now I shop based on what we need/want, not to stock up when I find options that are safe for him!

One thing I was most concerned about was making treatment work for him, especially with the rest period. My son is an active seven year old who is always moving. How could we possible expect him to rest for two hours every day? The reality has actually been better than I expected. We dose in the morning right after breakfast and before 7:00 a.m. His teacher knows he cannot run around or have PE before 9:00 a.m. Most of his rest period occurs while he is getting ready for school and being dropped off. I have a great picture that I love of him at the Great Wolf lodge lounging in a tube on the lazy river for the eleven minutes left of his rest period that occurred after the water park opened. It takes some time to figure out what works for you but the benefits so outweigh the annoyance that my son is much more on-board with the rest period than I ever expected.

SLIT and OIT for multiple food allergies with two children

Our first baby M started to have severe eczema at four months old, right when I returned to work after maternity leave. We had joined a nanny share and, unbeknownst to us, had chosen a nanny with messy snacking habits. M's eczema worsened over my first two months back at work. Her skin was seeping, and her urine output decreased to where there were crystals in her diapers. Our pediatrician prescribed topical steroids and suggested we switch from supplementing breast milk with standard milk formula to soy formula. Neither seemed to help.

With ongoing worsening eczema, we went to our first allergist when M was six months. Skin prick tests were positive for multiple foods (dairy, egg, wheat, soy, peanut, tree nuts, coconut), as well as dog. We were given the "I'm so sorry," avoid all these foods on the list, get rid of your dog, good luck and come back for retesting in six months speech. There was a brief period of relief thinking we had found a solution to fixing M's skin and making her more comfortable. Sadly, avoiding these foods (and our dog for two weeks) did not help her skin, and we continued putting mittens on her day and night while simultaneously worrying about her fine motor skills development. In hindsight, we believe that the culprit of her inability to heal was a combination of things: she was also allergic to sesame (not yet tested), and her skin was so bad after months of eczema that she needed a more aggressive treatment plan. I made the difficult decision to cut my work time in half, and we got a new nanny dedicated to only our child so that foods and the constant rubbing and itching could be monitored closely.

During this time, we were feeling very isolated with our frustration and sorrow. Combined with lack of sleep, I often felt panicky and afraid. As M approached eight months, I went to see a naturopath who cut my diet to just chicken, rice, beans, spinach, tomatoes, salt, and pepper. We experimented with different creams she'd given us (one contained sesame!). After a couple months of no improvement, she concluded the skin issues were not due to food and suggested we slowly open up our diets, including dairy. One evening, we decided to test two ounces of dairy formula. M became lethargic afterward. When we undressed her to change for bedtime, her entire body was red with hives starting to appear. I remember utter panic on both our parts. We put steroid cream all over her before we realized it was time to use epinephrine. We called 911, as we were told to do, yet were chastised when help arrived because she seemed just fine by that time. I am so grateful we went to the ER, as she had a second reaction upon arriving and needed another dose of epinephrine. At this point, the true realization set in: it wasn't just that our baby was itchy and uncomfortable all the time; she could also die.

When M was one, we scheduled an appointment to see our second allergist. He retested and confirmed all previous allergies plus sesame. We asked about oral challenges to give M more eating options. He felt that coconut and soy were the two allergens that were mild enough per the skin test that we could choose to trial at home. But he declined challenging the others, as they were too severe. This was a pretty low point for me.

I was very grateful for the coconut and soy additions, but I envisioned a future of home schooling, limited social gatherings, and isolation from the life I wanted for my child. I found myself in research mode and came upon the term OIT and found Dr. Jain.

Our second occurrence of anaphylaxis was the day before our first consult with Dr. Jain, when M was seventeen months old. We were getting ready to make the three-hour drive to stay in a hotel for an early morning appointment, and my husband pulled out a soy breakfast patty from the freezer to eat. M asked for a bite and he gave her one tiny bite. About an hour later, as we were getting M in the car, I noticed the skin around her eyebrows were dark red. Then the rest of her body followed. The horror and panic were back as I realized what was happening. She became more lethargic. This time we did not hesitate to give epinephrine. She immediately threw up, getting out the egg and milk that was in the soy patty. We called 911 and again went to the hospital.

Once we started SLIT, the stress and worry continued, but there was a light at the end of the tunnel that made life feel more bearable. It took us seven months to get to SLIT maintenance. My husband worked on Saturdays, allowing us to make the drive on Sundays for our Monday morning appointments. Weekly updoses were too much for M's body, so we changed to every other week and flew through the rest of the protocol. We immediately started food challenges after being on SLIT maintenance for a month. Stress and nerves for me every week—but it was worth it!

At age two, M had an amazing understanding that she would get to eat more foods if she passed the challenges and ate like a champ whatever was put into her cup of applesauce. We "passed" every challenge until we got to dairy, meaning M left the office having gotten to the end of the protocol without reacting. However, after both egg and peanut, she had symptoms on the drive home. With egg, her eczema flared up all over her body, and Dr. Jain stayed in contact with us as it resolved with multiple Zyrtec doses. Peanut was more severe. M's eczema was even more widespread on her body, and her eyes swelled up.

We didn't expect M to pass the dairy challenge, but we wanted to find out what our starting point for OIT should be. As predicted, we had to stop on just the first step. We waited until M was over two and a half before starting OIT, about six months after finishing food challenges. Although we were anxious to begin OIT, it was both hard work and exciting to get all the foods M had passed into her diet at least twice a week. Dairy OIT brought more stress and anxiety, and I was also pregnant with our second child. It was not smooth sailing, but we got through it. One incident that will always stay with me is the morning M seemed to be super tired and slept in well past her normal waking time. Dr. Jain advised us to skip the morning dose (standard dosing was twice a day at the time). As she was trying to eat breakfast, she vomited. We were back in contact with Dr. Jain, and he helped us make a plan to resume her dose at a decreased amount once she felt better and increase slowly to get back to her previous level. We have no clue what caused her reaction; once we got back on track, we didn't have any other major incidents.

M graduated from dairy OIT three months after new baby E was born and two months after my dad passed away. E started having the same eczema issues as M at four months old. Although I was deeply saddened that my second child likely also had food allergies, I thought I had a plan. We immediately got skin tests and a long list of foods to avoid (including dairy, egg, soy, peanuts, tree nuts as well as things like tomatoes and green beans). I stopped nursing and changed to an elemental/hypoallergenic formula. The skin did not improve. Dr. Jain's office referred us to a dermatologist, who had us implement a plan that was clearly written out and explained. That, along with starting SLIT, psychologically improved my outlook on life. If I were to compare M's journey to E's, I would say M suffered for much longer and more severely. As a parent trying to maneuver, though, I feel it was much worse for me with E. I felt I should know what I was doing, but the stress and worry had been ongoing for years by that time, and I don't think I could handle as much. E took about five months to get through SLIT, passed all food challenges except egg, took about six months for egg OIT, and now we are an allergy free family!

We owe the world to Dr. Jain and his staff. SLIT and OIT were definitely the right choices for us. I understand it might not be for everyone.

Our goal was to have our kids be able to life "normal lives" and not live in fear or feel like exclusion was the norm. My advice to parents is to research what is right for your family and involve other providers in your journey: dermatologist, dietitian, therapist/psychologist. Looking back, I can see the wisdom in having a treatment team to help all aspects of wellness, but when I was immersed in the allergy life, I was just trying my best and didn't get a chance to clearly assess our situation.

Post treatment, we are living life as I had originally envisioned. We're able to order from any restaurant (and eventually go out post-COVID). I am not packing a large bag of food "just in case" we get stuck in traffic or are out longer than expected, birthday parties when they resume will not be a source of anxiety, and both my kids can attend school with just the regular parent worries. We will continue blood tests each year to compare numbers. We will continue to incorporate the most severe allergens every day and the less severe ones at least twice a week. I still feel a bit uneasy whenever I see the girls scratching or being "tired" after meals, but I remind myself of how things were for them as babies and how I felt daily back then. To say SLIT and OIT were life changing is an understatement for our family.

SLIT and OIT for multiple food allergies and environmental allergies with two children

My daughter S struggled with severe eczema as a baby. She was almost exclusively breastfed, and we had taken her to dermatologists and allergists, and her skin prick tests came back negative. When S was one, we gave her yogurt at a family party, and she had a severe reaction with hives and swelling. We went to see an allergist, did another skin prick test, and this time dairy was definitely positive. Peanut was mildly reactive but not enough to be considered positive, and tree nuts were negative. We were prescribed epinephrine and were given general information about allergies and directions to strictly avoid dairy. I wasn't aware of how serious S's allergies were and that they were possibly life threatening.

An allergist in our family recommended we do an oral challenge at home to peanut, which led to our discovery that S was also severely allergic to peanut. We went back to the allergist, and he had a more serious talk with us about the possibility of anaphylaxis and how to parent a child with life-threatening allergies. We talked about how to read food labels and heard stories about reactions from cross-contact. We went home, purged our house of peanuts and tree nuts, and started paying more attention to labels. We resigned ourselves to no longer eating in restaurants.

Over the next few months, we noticed minor contact reactions due to cross-contamination with dairy, which my husband and I had continued to eat. Birthday parties were another source of reactions, and by the time she was two, we started leaving when the food was served. It was stressful to be around people eating and thinking about who had touched what with their nutty milky hands and the risks to my daughter. For the next several years, I hosted all the play dates and prepared all the food for family events so I could control it and make it safe for my daughter.

By the time S was three, we had a son, P, who we discovered also had a peanut allergy. Based on S's testing results, our allergist said it did not look like she would outgrow her dairy allergy on her own. He introduced us to the concept of OIT and told us about a doctor he knew who is a pioneer in OIT. He recommended we go talk to him and see if OIT was something we would want to pursue.

We set up a consultation with Dr. Jain, and he was very realistic about laying out the work that is involved with OIT, for the child, parents, and all the caretakers. When it came down to it, we were already doing a lot of hard work. We were already limiting social contact, being really careful with where we went, whom we saw, and what we ate. The amount of paperwork and interviews and groundwork I had to do to find a preschool and make sure they were following safety protocols was enormous. What Dr. Jain was proposing did sound like a lot of work, especially in the beginning, but the payoff was that if it worked, you would have a whole lot less work to do later, and that sounded really rewarding to us. He was also very reassuring about severe and long-term side effects and told us that a lot of that happens when you try to push things too much.

Since S was three years old, we thought it was worth asking her what she thought. Although young, she knew the life of an allergic person and could understand what OIT would look like and what we would have to do. She said let's do it.

When we started our OIT journey, it was just S because P was still too young. It meant taking time off work and putting off fully resuming my career so we could prioritize treatment. It was a once a week, full day commitment for us. I would pack food, clothes, toys, and entertainment in a suitcase, and we would drive forty-five minutes each way with no traffic to Dr. Jain's office. With traffic it could take up to an hour and a half. I was terrified during the first dose of diluted milk, but it was easier than I expected it to be. S was cooperative with getting her vitals taken and taking her doses. The first year of her doing OIT, I didn't have to bring any kind of screens or devices. I would read to her, and we would sing and draw. It was actually a special time that I look back on fondly.

We started experiencing some setbacks when we got to a 50 percent milk dilution. We started at age three and a half, and I had hopes she would be cleared for baked milk by her fourth birthday, but that didn't happen. Around her fourth birthday, she seemed to be reaching a plateau. We decided to keep dairy where it was and start peanut OIT. We started both S and P on peanut at about the same time. Having two kids in one room was definitely more challenging, and P was more active than S. They entertained each other, I started allowing TV, and I am eternally grateful to my mom, who helped us make appointments work.

Overall, my kids were fairly compliant, and Thursday OIT was our adventure for two years. When they were about halfway through, the taste became more significant, and they started fighting it. We had some difficult times getting them to take their doses, and it was definitely not always pleasant. I think the body naturally rejects anything the person is allergic to. Plus, if you've almost died from eating something, you will have a visceral reaction to the taste of that food. It was challenging to find things that would allow the right amount of protein without having to eat too much of the food so they would not gag all the time.

At one point, S hit a plateau with both dairy and peanut OIT and was not making progress. Rather than pushing ahead with those, we decided to start SLIT for tree nuts. Her tree nut allergies were not as severe as the dairy and peanut, and she was able to freely eat some tree nuts already. The hope was that SLIT for tree nuts would get her to the point of being able to eat foods with possible cross-contamination. Dr. Jain told us that SLIT would be easier in terms of long-term maintenance versus OIT. She was already having one-half cup of milk, twice a day, and would soon have five peanuts, once or twice a day. The thought of adding five nuts of each tree nut on top of that was too much; it would be an entire meal just of OIT doses.

We had no problems with SLIT; it was easy and went smoothly. We didn't have to fight the natural hatred of the food since she couldn't taste the nuts in the SLIT dose at all. We started SLIT and then went back to building up for dairy so we were doing both each week at our appointments. We utilized the same strategy for P. He went through peanut OIT pretty quickly and didn't hit a plateau. Like his sister, he could tolerate some tree nuts but not all (and different ones from her, of course). So we did SLIT after he graduated from peanut OIT. By the time he was getting to SLIT maintenance, S had graduated dairy OIT, was on SLIT maintenance for tree nut, and was getting really close to graduation for peanut OIT.

That was when Dr. Jain sat us down and told us that the next thing we had to tackle was environmental allergies. They were not old enough to be able to tolerate allergy shots, so he suggested doing SLIT for seasonal allergies. What he said is that, while allergy shots are the most effective thing you can do, you can use SLIT to get ahead so that, when you start shots, you can build up faster, and you don't have to do it for as long. The kids were familiar with the process of SLIT, so it was smooth.

Travelling with all the allergy stuff was definitely a challenge and interesting. I had a conversion chart with all the different kinds of dairy and brands S could have. For the peanuts, we just had to travel with ground up peanut everywhere we went. Plus the SLIT bottles, the EpiPens, and asthma inhalers.

S graduated from milk OIT at about four and a half. By the time she was five, she had graduated peanut OIT. P was done with peanut OIT by the time he was three. The last thing we did was oral challenges for tree nuts for both kids. If they could pass the oral challenges, all I would need to do was give them tree nuts twice a week to maintain that level of desensitization. They passed, and it was really exciting for all of us, a huge victory. Now I keep chocolate-covered cashews and walnuts in the house, and I give them to them a couple times a week. They are able to have crushed walnuts in baked goods and cookies. They don't love the taste of them, but they can tolerate them and it keeps them safe.

During the course of OIT updosing and postgraduation, we experienced some setbacks, mostly due to illness, but there were some unexpected setbacks as well. One of the unexpected challenges was what happens when little kids lose their baby teeth. It leaves a hole and allows the dose to go directly into the bloodstream, which can cause a major reaction. We had a really big scare when S lost her first tooth. We gave her milk dose that evening, and she blew up right in front of our eyes. Luckily, we had Dr. Jain's cell phone on speed dial and called him. It was a really big scare. Afterward, we had to lower her dose for a few days and build back up in the office. Subsequent tooth losses got progressively less traumatic, and dairy caused the biggest problem because milk is liquid and runs all over the mouth, whereas peanut is solid. The kids have had the flu, hand-foot-mouth, thrush, and, throughout, we've kept up with OIT and never had to stop it, only take steps back.

Now they are ten and eight. After they graduated, we went to Disneyland, and we bought them everything in the park. We went to all the restaurants, all the amusement parks. We traveled on an airplane, and we went to Hawaii last year. We've just had a really great few years. Like I said before, they've had all sorts of illnesses. I am really glad we were well past graduation when COVID hit because I can't imagine trying to do OIT during COVID time. I'm sure it's doable; it's just a lot of stress. I feel for the kids, because they had a few years of freedom, and now the world is on lockdown again. They didn't get to fully enjoy that freedom, but our hope for the future is that everyone can enjoy freely again.

SLIT, OIT, Chinese Herbs, and biologics for multiple food allergies and environmental allergies

At six years old, our son R can eat out at restaurants, sleep through the night, spend the night at friends' houses on his own, and go to birthday parties without us attending (and he can eat the cake!), but it wasn't always this way.

R had reactions to the food I ate while breastfeeding him and eczema that developed when he was about six weeks old. When he was old enough to try food and get allergy testing, we realized that he was a severe case. By about two years old, he had a very limited safe diet with confirmed allergies to tree nuts, peanuts, wheat, egg, dairy, sesame, soy, garlic, and some others; debilitating eczema; and he had been in the ER a few times for asthma. As parents of him (and by then also a newborn), our lives were very much led by fear, an abundance of caution, and zero spontaneity in our lives. Even as our careful, limited family lives were controlled by caring for our son, he had multiple food allergy reactions.

At two and a half years old, he began OIT for tree nuts. This first attempt at OIT was not very successful, and after six months of eczema flares, digestive issues, temper changes, and no OIT progress, we decided to stop OIT and begin SLIT for tree nuts and peanuts. About six months later, R had a severe anaphylactic reaction to an accidental ingestion of a small amount of baked powdered milk. After consulting with Dr. Jain, we decided to start OIT for dairy and egg because the world seemed to be too dangerous for our son. At that time, R was about three years old, and he had also become a patient of Dr. Li. Dr. Li's Traditional Chinese Medicine (TCM) work with our son initially focused on calming his system and his severe eczema. Her work with R, which has continued for four years, has led to his eczema and itching totally clearing up and all of his digestive issues being controlled. I do not believe that R would have been able to tolerate OIT without Dr. Li's TCM work, and we are so grateful for Dr. Jain's support of our combined efforts.

Over the next three years, R was on SLIT maintenance for tree nuts and peanuts; TCM with Dr. Li; and slowly worked toward OIT maintenance for wheat, dairy, egg, tree nuts, and peanuts. It was a challenging process, but it progressed. As he got closer to maintenance, he began to have some stomach pain, digestive issues, and more asthma flares with viruses, so Dr. Jain added Xolair to our treatment plan. After three months of Xolair (and continued TCM and SLIT), we were able to get our son to a low-level maintenance dose for peanuts, tree nuts, dairy, and egg. Now at seven years old, R continues to have once or twice daily OIT doses; SLIT for environmental allergens and tree nuts; monthly Xolair; and TCM treatment. He eats wheat and baked dairy and egg freely, can eat small amounts of soy (mainly in packaged goods), and can have foods that "may contain tree nuts and peanuts." His eczema has been gone for years, and his asthma is very well controlled. Our future goals are to complete environmental allergy shots and possibly build up his maintenance OIT doses to allow him more free eating. At the moment, R is comfortable and happy with what he can eat, and his food allergies don't feel very restrictive to us. We are comfortable calling ahead to restaurants and birthday parties and then sending him on his own to social events.

Dr. Jain has told us that R's case is unique and severe. It has been a long road logistically and emotionally for our whole family. All the treatments (SLIT, OIT, Xolair, and TCM) to treat his multiple food allergies, eczema, and asthma take a lot of planning and organization. My partner and I are both teachers, and around the beginning of our son's treatment and younger child's birth, I stopped working, in no small part to be available for organizing and facilitating treatment. The treatment has been emotional because, while we have complete access to Dr. Jain at all hours (and have called him many, many times), OIT treatment in particular requires caregivers to assess small "side effects" (or reactions) daily. In addition, requiring that a three year old eat complete portions of food they don't like twice per day, at the same times each day and within twenty minutes, was very challenging. We never considered stopping the treatment because we knew that it was the only way for our son to have a more normal life. That said, advice we'd give now for parents would be to have one parent with a flexible job, rally emotional support from friends and family, and anticipate incorporating emotional therapy into your lives.

We are now at a place where we live free, relaxed, more spontaneous lives. The stress and anxiety my partner and I felt since R was a baby remained through much of the treatment but, in the past two years, has lifted. Our son doesn't remember the limitations his life had in his early years or much of the challenges of the OIT updosing time. His current maintenance treatments are part of his daily life. At seven years old, he accepts them as part of his routine, much like daily tooth brushing. We are so grateful that we found Dr. Jain and that he and his staff have been willing to work with us through these years. Dr. Jain's treatments are totally tailored to each patient's needs and Dr. Jain takes caregiver's experience and goals seriously. We could not be more grateful to Dr. Jain and know that our son's current safety and freedom in the world is thanks to his attention and care for our son and family.

Chapter 12:

Psychological Considerations and Decision-Making

Up until now, you've primarily heard the voice of the first author and the first Elizabeth. In this last chapter, the narration and voice shift to the second Elizabeth. I am a licensed clinical psychologist who specializes in anxiety in children and adolescents. My orientation to therapy is heavily influenced by an approach called Acceptance and Commitment Therapy (ACT). ACT emphasizes making space for uncomfortable emotions and thoughts—and the pain that comes along with them—to exist. Rather than engaging in a battle to try to control those, you can instead choose to commit to leaning into present moment actions based on what is important to you to live a full and meaningful life.

My background and professional development were fortuitous after my second daughter was born in 2008. Within weeks, she developed severe eczema and seemed itchy and miserable most of the time. She pulled and scratched at her skin so much that we started taping socks to her hands and had to treat secondary bacterial infections from the wounds she inflicted on herself if her hands were not covered. She pulled her hair out, neither of us got much sleep, and she struggled to gain weight. We saw a series of dermatologists who prescribed increasingly higher doses of steroid creams and medications. I was exclusively breastfeeding her and asked each doctor we consulted whether or not I should be concerned that she might be reacting to something I was eating. Each one assured me that this was not food-related and that food proteins were too large to pass through breastmilk.

As was the recommendation at the time, we waited until six months of age to introduce solid foods and then slowly and carefully introduced one food at a time. We had done this with her older sister a few years earlier, and it went quite smoothly. My younger daughter had her first anaphylactic reaction at six months old. The only food she had ingested was pureed pears, but she was sitting at a table with adults who were eating a meal containing peanuts and sesame. I had never seen a severe allergic reaction before, and it took me a few minutes to even realize what was happening as she broke out in full body hives, and her face, eyes, mouth, and tongue swelled. We called the on-call pediatrician and left multiple messages with the answering service but did not receive a response for almost two hours. Even though the adults present included multiple medical and health care professionals, none of us realized how serious her condition might be. By the time the pediatrician called us back, she had exhausted herself and fallen asleep, and the danger seemed to have passed. We followed up with our pediatrician the next day and were given the advice to avoid pears and to buy some Benadryl.

She continued to have allergic reactions ranging from mild to more serious. Hives and minor swelling were a routine part of daily life from cross-contamination of foods we did not yet realize were problematic. When we introduced a new food (only during business hours) and she had a more serious reaction, we went to the pediatrician. At the time, these were not considered anaphylactic because her breathing did not seem impacted, but they would meet current criteria based on having two or more systems involved. These reactions commonly included full body hives, intense itchiness, facial edema, and vomiting. After each reaction, we were told to avoid that specific food and wait a few months before trying to reintroduce it. No one mentioned allergies or the need for epinephrine. At each visit, I asked for a referral for an allergist, and I was told it was not warranted.

After a few months of this, and having stopped trying to introduce new foods out of fear of what might happen, I fired our pediatrician and found a local allergist on my own. We still had no idea the severity of what we were dealing with. After many rounds of skin testing, she was diagnosed with allergies to more than a dozen different foods including seven of the nine top allergens. Testing was based on what foods we had already tried, as well as those one might commonly feed a ten month old with no teeth. As she got older and had new reactions, additional testing revealed more allergies. In addition, at almost three years old, she had an anaphylactic reaction after playing in the ocean and was diagnosed with cold-induced urticaria. A few years later, both of my daughters began having allergic reactions to the sun. So in addition to food allergies, asthma, and eczema, we also learned to prevent and manage allergic reactions caused by just about any climate we might encounter.

Psychological Control and Flexibility

At the same time that we were trying to determine what was happening with my daughter during the first year of her life, my mother was experiencing confusing symptoms and rapidly deteriorating health from what we soon would learn was early-onset dementia. Having these two experiences occur simultaneously challenged me on a deep level. The strategies I had relied on thus far in my life for dealing with problems were research, planning, and action, and my instinct was to jump in and get to work so I would feel more in control and less anxious. If my daughter only had one or even two allergies, this might have been the route I took. However, a hidden gift of her having so many and such severe allergies was that I knew I could not control the environment in a way that kept her safe, other than to never let her go anywhere outside our home. While that worked fairly well for an infant, it was not an ideal way for a child to develop and thrive longer term. The magnitude and complexity of how to keep her safe was so great that it freed my mind to have a different perspective and orientation.

As a child psychologist, I know that parents predominantly shape how a child views themself and the safety of the world. Extending that to food allergies, I realized I would be the most important model for how my daughter thought about this part of herself and what was and was not possible. I considered how I wanted her to see her allergies: as serious challenges to be managed with creative and flexible problem-solving. Something always present but not the totality of her identity or a limiting factor in exploring the world and living a full life. I visualized how I wanted her to grow up and imagined her as strong, brave, confident, and competent. And I thought about my older daughter, at that time four years old, and how she was experiencing her sister's allergies and the changes we were making as a family. Unlike my younger daughter, who did not yet have the language skills to truly understand, my older daughter did and I wanted to convey to her that these were manageable issues. With these values in mind, I worked backward on how to structure our daily life to support this mission.

I let go (mostly, on good days) of my desire for control and certainty and instead embraced a more realistic acceptance of our reality, risk management, and mindfulness about where to focus my energy and attention. I immersed myself in learning everything I could about food allergies. I walked the aisles of the supermarket like a library, picking up and reading each and every label. I made mental and written notes about what foods have which ingredients, what might be safe to try, and what substitutes might be available to replace the foods my four year old enjoyed but that were now unsafe to have around my one year old. I read cookbooks and online articles and developed new skills for making food attractive and appealing with limited ingredient options.

Over the years, I have tried to focus on what can be eaten, rather than what cannot, and convey a sense of abundance and possibility instead of deprivation. I intentionally tried to shift cultural messaging about the importance of food in gatherings and celebrations and actively emphasized the richness of connecting with people, having a good time, and building memories. One thing that aided this is that our extended family has a variety of different eating styles and needs. Many are vegetarian or pescatarian, and years later I was diagnosed with celiac disease and have to strictly avoid gluten. We have erred on the side of having more food and options than is necessary, so everyone is getting as much of the full meal experience as possible. Whenever we go to a party or outside gathering, I bring many different options for my daughter so she has choice and control over what she wants to eat. This has meant a lot of advanced preparation and a second freezer full of safe foods to pull from at a moment's notice, rather than avoiding a social event because of the lack of food options.

A big part of this shift toward greater psychological flexibility was accepting that allergic reactions would likely happen, despite the care we were taking to prevent them. Instead of becoming locked into the struggle to definitely prevent them, we leaned into the importance of practicing our emergency action plan and being prepared to implement it. As my daughter grew older, we worked with her on what was under her control and role-played how to handle difficult situations. We've talked a lot about values and how we approach hard things while loosening control about other people and outcomes. And we regularly practice injecting oranges with expired EpiPens so she is comfortable with the feel and process. While this has been instrumental for managing risk from allergies, it has also given her a sense of empowerment and control in making choices about treatment for her allergies.

This all sounds neat and tidy, and in reality, it has been anything but that. Like any new and hard mindset change, it was often two steps forward and one step back. I have experienced lots of doubt and fear and questioned my decisions. At times I got lost and reactive to anxiety, often caused by new developmental stages and dilemmas. The practice was and is to return to a place of acceptance that none of us can keep our children perfectly safe and that mistakes and pain are necessary for them to learn and grow and become resilient.

Managing Food Allergy Anxiety

Entering into the world of food allergies was overwhelming and brought with it fear about how to protect our little girl and ensure she stay healthy and safe. While some anxiety is absolutely necessary and adaptive with food allergies, I immediately understood the risk for both parents and children of developing a clinical anxiety disorder. Our first allergist gave me the advice early on to not fall into the trap of trying to control my daughter's environment as a means of managing her allergies and my anxiety. Instead, he said, invest my energy in training my daughter how to live in and navigate her environment. I saw the wisdom in this and took it to heart.

Throughout this book, we've talked about desensitization treatments for food allergies and the process of retraining your immune system. Managing and treating anxiety is very similar and shares quite a bit of the same terminology. Evidence-based treatment for anxiety includes what is known as exposure and response prevention, often done through the process of systematic desensitization. Those are clinical terms that mean that, instead of strictly avoiding the thing you are afraid of, you expose yourself to it in small steps and gradually build up tolerance. Like immunotherapy, the goal is to find the "just right" dose psychologically. It's an amount that is hard but doable with some stretching. Through repetition at that dose, a person expands their window of tolerance, and psychological flexibility increases and reactivity decreases.

This can be put into practice both in living with strict avoidance of allergens and in pursuing treatment where you are deliberately exposing your body to the allergen. Many children are terrified at just the thought of their allergen, let alone seeing it or coming into physical contact with it. I've treated a number of kids who have developed anxiety disorders because they cannot control what everyone else is doing around them. While their home and even classroom might be allergen-free, the homes of their extended family and friends are not, their school is not, playgrounds are not, and the larger world is not. They might become so scared that they stop wanting to go anywhere for fear they might encounter their allergen. Or they develop compulsive behaviors to cope with the anxiety and over time these grow and begin impacting their functioning. Just the thought of the food has become synonymous with possible death and is terrifying.

Most kids with food allergies will not have a serious reaction unless the allergen actually gets inside their body. So, treatment for anxiety might involve a series of steps whereby they get increasingly closer and closer to the allergen and learn how to calm themselves in the presence of it while taking concrete strategies to keep themself safe. For example, they might progress from being in the same room as the allergen, to looking at it from a few feet away, to inspecting it up close or even holding it briefly and then immediately washing their hands. In the context of a patient engaged in food allergy treatment, the next step might include putting the food into their mouth and swallowing a small amount. This is done, of course, in close collaboration with the allergist to ensure that these actions are safe for the child. Treating anxiety gives a child a stronger sense of control of their emotional reaction and a more balanced perspective on fear, so the world feels a little less scary.

More often than not, parents need these strategies and coaching long before their children do. Children absorb the energy and messages (both direct and indirect) given by caregivers. Food allergy parents have to manage a lot of anxiety-provoking situations and make individual decisions that are best for them about what level of risk is acceptable and ways to mitigate that risk. They might communicate through facial expression and words how scary the world is to their young child. They might fixate on how to control the environment and other people to make it safe for their child. They might want to avoid playgrounds, restaurants, birthday parties, and holiday celebrations totally because of the emotional and physical work involved. Or they might go the other direction and embrace "normal" life without enough thought and consideration to risk. Some people try to not feel anxiety by avoiding or controlling the situations that provoke it, and some deal by pushing it down and denying its existence.

As a food allergy parent and psychologist, I've witnessed the full gamut of emotional experiences that accompany this condition. I'm not saying that every scary situation should be faced head-on and tackled or that it's wrong to modify environments and routines for safety. Rather, as parents we need to be mindful of our own emotional reactions and thoughtful about what messages we send our children about living with food allergies. This starts at a young age, before they are able to understand our words and explanations. Maintaining a calm facial expression and moving young children out of harm's way is key. As is communicating in a matter-of-fact tone of voice and setting clear limits. We can express understanding and empathy and also communicate that it's okay to feel afraid and still engage in important activities of daily life. After all, while avoidance of feeling anxious might bring short-term relief, it often leads to long-term loss of vitality and opportunity. It is essential that our children learn how to show up and do hard things throughout their lives; dealing with food allergies can help them learn this lesson early on.

Healthy Emotional Development

Childhood is filled with important developmental tasks, and I'd like to highlight a few that are especially relevant to children with food allergies. In the earliest years, children are learning whether they can trust caregivers to reliably take care of them and whether or not the world is a fundamentally good and safe place. Children then go on to developing a sense of mastery and competence, a feeling that they are able to successfully navigate their world and can connect action and consequence. As they move into later childhood and adolescence, emotional work centers more on independence and identity development.

Encouraging Mastery and Competence

As we moved out of infancy and into the toddler years with my daughter, I was thinking about these developmental tasks of childhood. I focused my energy and control on structuring her home and school environments in ways that supported her being as independent and "normal" as possible. This involved some of the following:

- A thorough reorganization of our pantry and refrigerator to clearly identify with color stickers safe and unsafe foods.

- Allowing her to choose her own snacks from the safe foods.

- Giving her language to talk about how her body feels and teaching her how to tune in, listen, and trust her body and its signals.

- Involving her in food preparation and talking about ingredients and nutrition from an early age.

- Developing a system with her preschool teacher and the other classroom parents to quickly tag lunches as safe or unsafe (in our case, this was around messy allergens that were likely to spill or smear).

- Allowing her to eat at the same table with a child eating her allergens as long as they were not the messy ones.

- Developing really good practices around not touching her nose or mouth, not putting things into her mouth, and hand washing.

- Keeping spare food in the classroom that she can access on her own in case her food drops or gets contaminated in some way.

- Keeping treats at school for those inevitable surprise desserts that show up in the classroom without advance warning.

A key part of all of this was how I communicated about the precautions. I tried to keep a calm, matter-of-fact voice and facial expression and convey how manageable the situation was. Even when she was young, I would share in appropriate ways what I might be concerned about and how we might address it, giving her choices whenever I could. I would ask for her ideas and try to incorporate them as much as possible so she would have a sense of control over her experience. We talked through problem-solving and decision-making together.

Even though she was never without a parent or trusted caregiver in those early years, it was important to me that she grow up with the unquestionable routine of taking her "go bag" with her and communicating about her allergies. We called it a go bag because it went everywhere she did. I did not want to establish the routine of relying solely on an adult to hold the knowledge and tools for her safety and make this invisible to her. Rather than throwing EpiPens into a plastic baggy in my purse, I had bags custom made in bright fun fabrics that were large enough to fit all the necessities and had a loop and small carabineer on the outside. Our go bag can be thrown into a larger bag, or it can be clipped onto something (such as a belt loop, bike, water bottle, etc.). We leave the go bag by the front door and make a point of grabbing it as part of our leaving the house routine. After years of repetition, taking the go bag is now as natural as putting on shoes before walking out the door. As my daughter got older, we transferred responsibility to her for carrying it when we're out. An enticement for this has been finding cute bags that fit her go bag and snacks. She has an extensive collection and love for handbags and enjoys matching her bags to her outfit, mood, and the needs of the outing.

Our go bag is stocked with the medications my daughter might need, as well as a food allergy card (a business card with a cute design and her picture, allergies, and emergency action plan, including phone numbers, on the back). We updated the cards as she got older and allowed her to pick the design. As a young child, we ordered enough that she could carry and share them with whomever she wanted. My older daughter liked the cards so much, we made her ones too. They both delighted in handing out their cards and it made it a fun experience.

Something that was important to our family before allergies that we did not want to totally give up was travel and outdoor adventures. While allergies certainly impact where we go, what kind of accommodations we need, and our activities, we have found ways to explore the world. The mental pivot is how to anticipate and solve problems in advance. I plan out meals based on what foods I can reliably find and what shelf-stable items I can bring with us. I set aside my normal attention to healthy nutrition and variety and instead rely on easy-to-carry snacks and treats (aka, candy) that will fill her and allow us to be out for a full day. We set expectations that food might be repetitive and boring while traveling and talk about how this allows us to stay safe and focus on exploration, experiences, and memories. For sure, traveling brings a higher level of anxiety and requires more mindfulness and deep breathing than staying at home does. It has also been deeply enriching and helped to cultivate a mindset of exploration and competency.

Fostering Independence and Identity Development

At age thirteen, my daughter has outgrown many allergies, and she has developed new ones; we have successfully treated some, are in the process of treating others, and have acceptance that some may be with her for the foreseeable future. It is an ongoing process for all of us. As we enter into adolescence, I am leaning into the discomfort of allowing her to make more decisions for herself and not jumping in to tell her what to do and how to do it. Instead, as I've tried to do all along, I ask questions that get her brain thinking about what the concerns and potential challenges are. We try to brainstorm solutions and talk in terms of *how* and not *if*. There is openness, curiosity, and willingness to explore and experience all sorts of thoughts, feelings, and physical sensations. Rather than teaching her that discomfort always means something is wrong and needs to be eliminated, we sit with it and feel it with mindfulness.

As a parent, this has meant becoming more comfortable with allowing my daughter to struggle without trying to fix it for her and instead acting more as a consultant. Of course, there are limits, and it is still my responsibility to make sure she is as safe as possible. However, I push myself to allow her to make mistakes and learn from them whenever possible. In these preteen and teen years, it is our responsibility to encourage independence and autonomy in our children while keeping a solid safety net underneath them. And when they fall, as they inevitably will, we are there to love and support them and help them back onto their feet. This builds competence and resiliency.

Humans develop identity about who they are and who they are not. We have concepts about ourselves and can easily rattle off a list of "I am" statements that reflect both fixed characteristics and changeable qualities. Identity is related to experience and shapes our sense of self-worth and agency (the ability to have control over actions and their consequences). Identity formation is complex and is rapidly developing during childhood and adolescence.

For those with food allergies, this distinction potentially becomes an important part of their life experience and identity. It is something they carry with them everywhere and is part of many, if not all, major decisions they make. Most children with food allergies have felt the pain of being different from others and being left out of activities. They might also have experienced a sense of fear and helplessness about certain situations or the world more broadly. On the other hand, they might also experience a sense of specialness or uniqueness that comes with having food allergies. More likely than not, allergies and food have received a lot of attention throughout their lives, and some of this might be perceived positively, rather than negatively. All of these experiences contribute to a sense of identity and help answer the question "Who am I?"

For older children/adolescents, making the decision to pursue food allergy treatment might give rise to mixed thoughts and feelings about who they will be without having allergies in the same way. The spectrum runs from excitement and hope to fear, not only over the risks and challenges of treatment but also the issue of identity and not knowing what life without allergies is like. I heard this from my daughter when we discussed a treatment plan to target most of her allergies and she showed resistance. She poignantly said, "But allergies is what people know about me and makes me special." Food allergies have been one of the most consistent and defining features of her life, and we were talking about altering that. This opened up many wonderful conversations about what makes her special and the role of allergies in shaping who she is and who she wants to be in the world.

Another aspect of identity that relates to food allergy treatment is how to define yourself if you successfully get to free eating status with your allergen. How do you fill out forms asking about allergies? Do you still need to carry epinephrine with you at all times? Do you still need a 504 educational plan? These are all questions to answer in consultation with your allergist. We believe that, based on current understanding, most people with treated allergies need to continue to consider themselves at risk for having an allergic reaction and be prepared to treat it. While vigilance and caution are eased, they are not entirely removed. As more and more people successfully undergo treatment, as a society we need commonly understood terms and definitions to describe these situations.

Decision-Making

As you've read through this book and thought about your own family and situation, you are probably trying to decide whether or not to pursue treatment, which one might be right, how to stage it, and where to start. You might be intrigued about potential future treatments and wonder if you should hold off. The decision to wait for new treatments or use treatments that are currently available is a very personal decision. Existing food allergy treatments generally work really well for the simple cases that these new therapies would most likely treat, at least initially. And for the more complex cases, those not so easily treated with existing methods, these new treatments may not be available for quite a long time. When considering whether to treat now or wait, it is worth considering the years of freedom that can be gained by treating now. In addition to the quality of life impacts that food allergy treatments can have, there is also the possibility that desensitization can be passed on to future generations. The potential to alter the progression of food allergies is one the most interesting and compelling pieces of information for me in the decision-making process.

We would all like to think we can know what is going to happen in the future. The sense of control this gives us is important psychologically and is something we crave. The truth is, though, uncertainty is assured and lies down both the path of engaging in treatment and not engaging in treatment. Whatever choice you make, I encourage acceptance that you will not have a clear picture of what the outcome will be and instead make decisions based on the current best understanding of the state of treatment, probabilities, and your values for your child and family.

Choosing continued allergen avoidance is not without risk, both physically and emotionally. Living with food allergies takes a toll. And engaging in treatment has many costs associated with it, as well. While treatment may proceed smoothly and quickly, there are also often unforeseen twists and turns along the way, especially in more complicated cases. You will be served by being flexible and adapting to new information and needs as they arise. The writing of this chapter is occurring in the context of the COVID-19 pandemic, a situation that underscores this point about uncertainty and risk tolerance. It is helpful to consider the future and have goals, yet we can also know there are no guarantees, and we can make space for changes to occur.

If your child is older, including them in the decision-making process is an important consideration. In the case of my daughter, our first allergist was an early adopter of private practice OIT and talked to us about it from the very beginning. We had a tentative plan to start when she was about four years old and could more reliably tell us what she was experiencing. However, her reaching this stage coincided with the final months of my mother's life and then dealing with the aftermath brought by death. That, plus a host of other personal stressors, led us to hold off on starting formal OIT.

We were fortunate that, up until age six, my daughter had outgrown at least one major allergen each year, and finding safe foods/meals was becoming easier between that and the increasing availability of products for those with food restrictions. We were also able to use adapted OIT strategies to help accelerate desensitization at home to foods that seemed to be lessening in severity based on her annual testing. However, with each year, it was becoming clearer that many of her allergies would not be outgrown and she was adding new ones to the list. By the time the adults were ready to commit to OIT, my daughter was resistant and did not want to participate in treatment. She was fearful about reactions and the logistical complications of following the protocol. From her point-of-view, allergy avoidance was working just fine, she was enjoying her life, and OIT seemed difficult, burdensome, and risky. In particular, the maintenance phase of treating so many allergies, many of which she does not want to eat or it is cumbersome to eat on a daily basis, was daunting. Her ability to understand the long-term implications and payoff was limited, and the more we talked about it, the more opposed she became.

It wasn't until we moved and switched allergists to Dr. Jain that the option for SLIT became available. She was much more willing to engage in SLIT and successfully reached maintenance on dairy SLIT, passed a baked milk challenge and is doing baked milk OIT, and got to SLIT maintenance for tree nuts and a variety of other minor allergens. We also identified significant environmental allergies (she has no apparent symptoms) and started allergy shots. Once the pandemic is over, we still need to tackle her remaining severe allergies, as well as those that require customizable extracts. But the success she has had so far, and the overall positive experience, has led her to be more open to continuing treatment in the future.

As you explore and make decisions about what is right for your family, hold onto realistic expectations. There is fear in having allergies, there is fear in treating allergies, and there is fear in living with treated allergies. There is no living without fear. We are all vulnerable and at risk. Consider what your goals of treatment might be and what the treatment and maintenance protocols look like. Get emotional support and expand your social networks. Dealing with food allergies is hard work, and we all need help and support. Build upon and strengthen skills for managing discomfort, uncertainty, and anxiety. Focus on what matters to you as a family and what values you want to put at the center of your lives. Values are process and not outcome oriented. You can work toward them and live by them, whether or not you choose to engage in treatment. Remember that you are a mirror for your child's self-worth and competence. They learn to view themselves, their abilities, and the safety of the world through your eyes. There are no absolute right and wrong answers, and there are ways to support psychological flexibility and a growth mindset whichever path you choose.

Conclusion

I started thinking about and working on this book as my two children underwent food allergy treatments many years ago. I was struck by the lack of clear, easy to understand information available to families, and wanted to help fill that gap. The book has evolved and changed over the years from first concept to final revisions. I am hopeful that we have met my goal of providing high quality information about scientifically grounded treatment options and shared perspectives from multiple families that have chosen to undertake these treatments.

Any book like this captures information and understanding at a given point in time. We fully expect that the science of food allergy treatment will continue to progress. Current treatments will be modified and improved and new and exciting treatments will likely become available in the future. This is good news! We all benefit from ongoing clinical research and efforts of private practice allergists to refine the safety and effectiveness of protocols and expand access to treatment.

Our intention is not to influence you about one particular treatment or path. Rather, we want to give you the information you need to make informed choices. Your journey might parallel one of those highlighted here or go a different direction. We know that each family and situation is unique and only you can balance all the variables involved to make the best decision about if, when, and how to pursue food allergy treatment. All three of the authors have either personally been in this position as parents and/or helped guide people in the process. We know the suffering that comes with food allergies, and we know the complications and joys that come with treating those allergies and opening up new experiences and ways of life that were formerly closed off. Wherever your journey takes you, we wish you and your loved ones health, safety, and peace of mind.

Advice from a Food Allergy Dietitian

by Chau Brondan, MS, RD

I worked as an Intensive Care Unit (ICU) dietitian, and then I had two babies. Both developed severe food allergies, and I slowly transitioned to specializing in this in my career. At the beginning of our journey, many people imagined it was easy to handle my kids' severe food allergies with my background. While perhaps I had a leg up on other food allergy parents, food allergies had only been a short discussion during graduate school, and most of my critically ill patients in the ICU were on tube feeding. There was a lot to learn and after six years, I continue to learn along with patients and parents.

I am often asked questions about how to feed a child with food allergies. The short answer is that there is no one right way to do it. There are so many different combinations of allergies, ages, personalities, family dynamics and values, to name just a few variables. In addition, there are differences in access to stores and products based on geography and financial stability. The answer to this question is very specific and personal. And, as with everything with raising children, this topic takes time, patience, a lot of trial and error, and of course lots of love and understanding.

Here are some of the most common questions I get from parents of kids with food allergies:

- Is my child eating enough?
- Is my child eating a well-balanced diet?
- How do I get my child to eat more variety?

These are also common questions that parents of any children may ask! We are not so different in what we are seeking for our children, but the limitations that food allergies create can be extra daunting and stressful. Here are some general concepts that might help give parents of children with food allergies some peace of mind. There are three types of goals you can look at to help assess your child's food intake: measurable goals, visual goals, and intuitive goals.

Measurable goals would be such things as computing daily calories, number of servings of food groups, or grams of protein. You can do a web search for phrases such as "calorie needs for six year old boy" or "servings of dairy for four year old girl" to find acceptable ranges from respected institutes such as the National Institutes of Health or Cleveland Clinic. You'll see slight variations depending on the source, but generally they are split up between ages and by gender after the age of three and include calorie recommendations and goals for protein, fruit, vegetables, grains, and dairy intake. These recommendations are there for knowledge and as a general guideline. In my opinion, strict measurable goals are only necessary if there are indications of a deficit such as poor weight gain, poor growth, or lab work indicating micronutrient deficiencies.

In terms of visual goals, a good guideline is the healthy plate model. Regardless of allergy status, our meals should roughly be 50 percent non-starchy vegetables, 25 percent protein, and 25 percent grains. For younger kids, looking at intake over one to three days may be more realistic. There are many different versions of the healthy plate concept, the most common being the myplate.gov version. Visual goals are an approximation, and loosely estimating is ok. Consciously noting what your child is eating might trigger some realizations and insights about where improvements can be made. Keeping a journal of your child's intake (it does not need to include exact amounts) can be helpful for both parents and a dietitian to review.

Last are intuitive goals. When children are small, they are intuitive eaters: they eat when their bodies are hungry and stop when they don't feel hunger anymore. If an assessment shows no major concerns and parents agree, allowing children to eat intuitively (but still safely within their limitations) is an option. I discuss measurable goals and visual goals with parents to ensure they have the understanding of what is "ideal" in terms of adequate calories and appropriate food groups or appropriate division of vegetables, protein, and grains. Their goal is to present this ideal diet to the child but then step back and let the child make their own choices. Oftentimes with food allergies, meal times are marred by stress and negativity. A child might want something on your plate that they are allergic to; parents focus on "you have to eat this" or "you haven't eaten enough." Focusing on intuitive goals takes some of the pressure off both parents and children and gives the child a sense of control.

For families undergoing treatment for food allergies, working with a dietitian who specializes in this area is important and makes the process easier. Consider the example of a child who is incorporating egg and milk into their diet after SLIT or OIT and is directed to eat cupcakes multiple times a week. A dietitian assessing for general nutrition might not think eating sweets so often is beneficial and might not have a good understanding of allergy treatments, the need for regular exposure of the allergen prepared in controlled ways, and the complications of what other foods the child might need to eat for their treatment plan. I have spoken to a mom who shared her family was vegan, but even with lentil and several nut allergies, they did not wish to add animal products for protein. Another family grew all their foods and ate as "clean" as possible and only made the exception for a couple packaged snacks because of the limited foods that were safe to eat.

Finding a dietitian is like finding any other medical provider. It should be someone who assesses and advises but also listens and respects your family's personal beliefs and wishes. I believe that allergy treatments make my job easier. There is this light at the end of the tunnel that would not be there without these therapies. I find it more hopeful to discuss avoidance of allergens until treatment is completed, rather than forever. While the process is long and may not work for everyone and all foods, the joy of seeing someone move from avoidance to incorporating those foods into their daily diet is amazing and priceless.

Additional Resources

Websites

- American Academy of Allergy, Asthma & Immunology: https://acaai.org
- Food Allergy Research and Education (FARE): https://www.foodallergy.org
- Kids with Food Allergies: https://www.kidswithfoodallergies.org
- OIT 101: https://www.oit101.org

Books

- *Asthma, Allergies, Children: A Parent's Guide* by Henry Ehrlich, Paul Ehrlich, Larry Chiaramonte (2010).
- *The End of Food Allergy: The First Program to Prevent and Reverse a 21st Century Epidemic* by Kari Nadeau and Sloan Barnett (2020).
- *Food Allergies: A Complete Guide for Eating When Your Life Depends on It* by Scott Sicherer (2013).
- *The Food Allergy Fix: An Integrative and Evidence-Based Approach to Food Allergen Desensitization* by Sakina Shikari Bajowala (2018).

- *Food Allergies: Traditional Chinese Medicine, Western Science, and the Search for a Cure* by Henry Ehrlich (2014).
- *Kids Food Allergies for Dummies* by Mimi Tang and Katie Allen (2012).
- *Traditional Chinese Medicine, Western Science, and the Fight Against Allergic Disease* by Xiu-Min Li and Henry Ehrlich (2016).
- *Understanding and Managing Your Child's Food Allergies* by Scott Sicherer (2006).

About the Authors

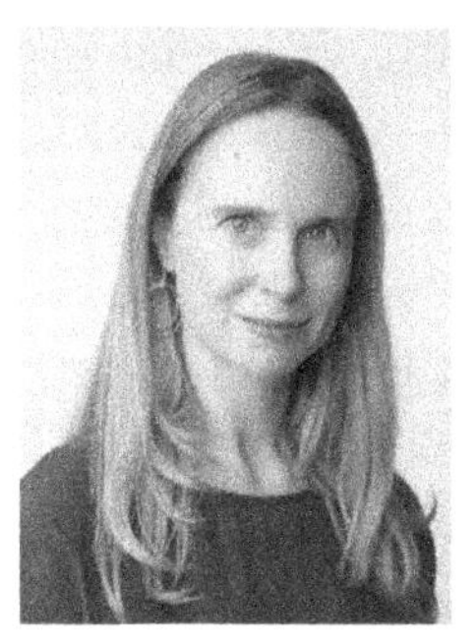

Elizabeth Muller

Elizabeth is the cofounder and CEO of Deep Isolation, a growing startup company that is working to solve the nuclear waste problem. She is also the cofounder and president of Berkeley Earth, a scientific research organization that focuses on environmental issues like global warming and air pollution.

Elizabeth is a mother to two children who suffered from severe food allergies, an eleven-year-old girl formerly allergic to peanuts, tree nuts, buckwheat, and fish, and a seven-year-old boy now consuming many of the forty-one foods he was previously allergic to—including milk/dairy, legumes, seeds, nuts, and fruits. Elizabeth has a unique perspective on food allergy treatments because she has had her own children use three out of the four major treatments currently available. Thus, she offers not only scientific understanding but also a unique perspective for parents who are seeking treatment but who don't yet know which treatment they want to pursue.

Thanks to her extensive research of the published scientific literature and discussions with leading experts, Elizabeth has become a leading contributor on social media for the topic of food allergy treatment. She is a Quora 2017 and 2018 "Top Writer" with more than 2 million views on her answers and over 27,000 followers. She is a "most viewed" writer on allergies with more than 100,000 views. She is also well known for the Facebook groups that she leads and participates in on food allergies and their treatments.

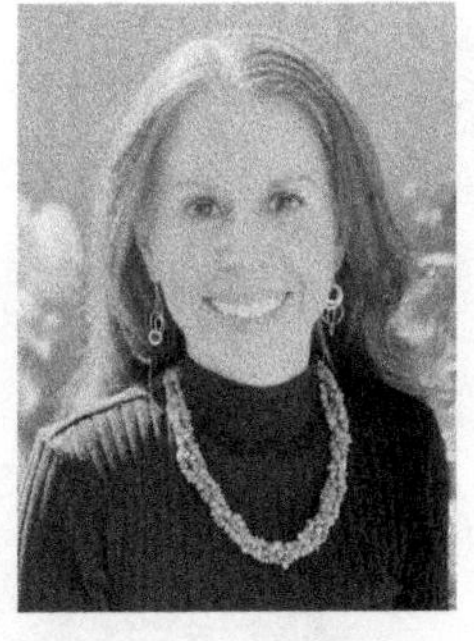

Elizabeth Hawkins, PhD MPH

Dr. Hawkins is a clinical psychologist, behavioral health consultant, and a food allergy mom and advocate. She holds a doctorate in child clinical psychology and an MPH in Health Services from the University of Washington. Dr. Hawkins is licensed and maintains a private therapy practice in the states of Washington and Oregon. One area of specialization is working with food allergy families to manage the accompanying stress, anxiety, and traumatic experiences that tend to occur with allergies.

Dr. Hawkins is also the mother of two children. Her youngest daughter was severely allergic to more than twenty different foods, including seven of the nine top allergens, and suffered from severe eczema and environmental allergies. Some of her allergies were outgrown, some have been successfully treated with two of the treatments described in the book and are now included in her daily diet, and she is currently undergoing treatment for others.

Dr. Hawkins combines her personal experience and education/training to help build and maintain emotional health and wellbeing for those living with food allergies. More information can be found at https://www.foodallergypsychologist.com

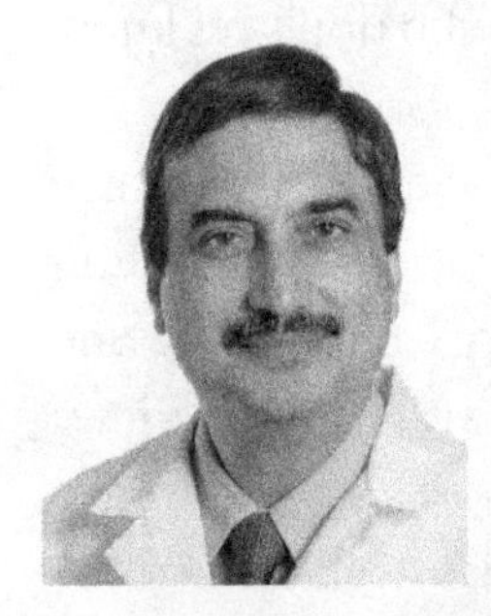

Sanjeev Jain, MD PhD

Dr. Jain was one of the first medical doctors to offer desensitization treatment in private practice and possibly the first to do combined tree nuts in a single protocol. Dr. Jain first received joint MD and PhD degrees from the University of Wisconsin and finished his residency at the University of Texas. He completed his advanced fellowship training in Allergy and Clinical Immunology at Yale University School of Medicine. He then taught and practiced at the University of Washington Medical School in Seattle, where he developed a reputation as one of the finest allergists in the region. He has won numerous awards and is included in the Guide to America's Top Physicians consistently for the last several years.

As an allergist, Dr. Jain treasures the opportunity to witness his patients make dramatic improvements after years of suffering. He can recall several instances where his patients who had previously required repeated hospital admissions for asthma exacerbations, food allergy reactions, and other medical conditions, have returned to normal lives free of hospital visits. In Dr. Jain's experience, most patients can achieve significant improvements by determining the individual triggers of their allergic reactions and by instituting appropriate therapy.

Dr. Jain's practice, Columbia Allergy, has twelve clinic locations in the states of California, Oregon, Washington, and Idaho. More information can be found at https://columbiaallergy.com

CPSIA information can be obtained
at www.ICGtesting.com
Printed in the USA
BVHW061523200223
658844BV00016B/1084

9 798885 900218